Mental Health

Edited by
Rob Garbett, RGN, BN

Illustrated by
Peter Gardiner

 **NT** *books*

emap BUSINESS COMMUNICATIONS

Published by
Emap Healthcare, part of Emap Business Communications Ltd
Greater London Road,
Hampstead Road
London NW1 7EJ

Companies and representatives throughout the world
Film output (repro) by Prepress Services, Leeds, West Yorkshire
Printed in Great Britain by Drogher Press, Christchurch, Dorset

ISBN 1 902499 20 4

Contents

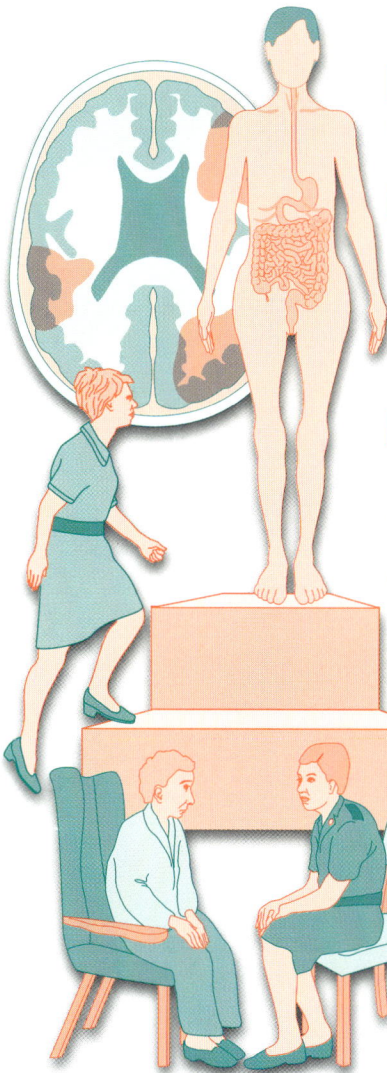

CONTRIBUTORS

Eating disorders:
Authors: Christine Halek, BA, RMN, senior nurse practitioner (parts 1-3); Denis Cremin, RMN, DipN, nurse practitioner (part 1); Beverley Murphy, RMN, nurse practitioner (part 3) all at Annexe Nursing Development Unit, Pathfinder NHS Trust, London

Schizophrenia:
Author: Julie Repper, MPhil, BA, RGN, RMN, research student, Manchester University

Depression:
Author: Elizabeth Armstrong, RGN, RHV, mental health development officer, Institute of Psychiatry, London

Dementia:
Author: Lynne Phair, BSc, RMN, RGN, DPNS, MIFA, team leader, Mental Health Services for Older People, Eastbourne and County Health Care NHSTrust, Seaford, East Sussex

PROFESSIONAL DevelopmeNT

Keep yourself up to date

Use your reading as a vital part of your professional updating

Welcome to *Nursing Times'* Professional Development Book 5. It follows on from our popular Professional Development *Nursing Times* series (PDNT), which ran for over three years.

The contents have been revised and updated to ensure that they reflect contemporary thinking in the areas concerned. The books are designed for busy clinical nurses looking to update their knowledge and skills, for students and for practitioners returning to work after a break.

Each unit concludes with a multiple choice questionnaire for you to test your knowledge. This book and others in the series provide you with one means to keep up to date and relate your learning practice so that you can meet the UKCC's standards for post registration education (PREP).

This book uses *Nursing Times* Study Hours help you keep a record of what you learn and how long it took you.

PROFESSIONAL DevelopmeNT

PREP MADE SIMPLE

Lifelong learning is an important part of every nurse's working life. The UKCC has provided a framework to help nurses relate their learning to practice in order to provide safe and effective practice.

While there has been a degree of anxiety about how to meet the minimum requirement of five days study or its equivalent, we at *Nursing Times* believe that reading the professional press can be of great help.

Study Hours have been designed by *Nursing Times* to provide an easy-to-use estimation of the time you spend reflecting on and studying clinical issues. Using Study Hours puts you in control of your own professional development and helps you meet the PREP requirements.

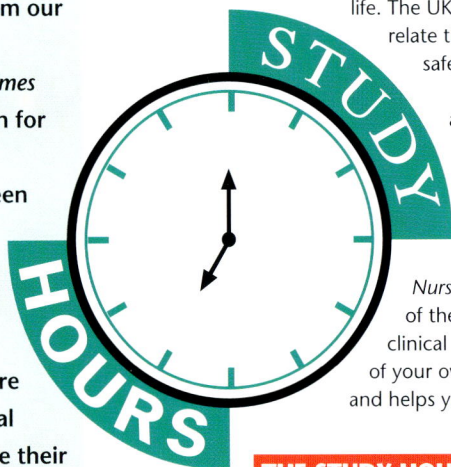

THE STUDY HOURS RATING

The Study Hours rating is the figure inside the clock. It is our estimate of the number of hours it will take you to read and reflect on the material provided.

The figure given is our estimate but it does not matter if you take more or less time; record the time you spend in your professional profile.

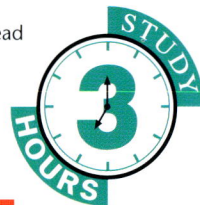

STUDY HOURS IN PRACTICE

Reading articles, supplements and publications such as this can be a passive affair but it can also, if you choose, be the starting point of a great deal of reflection and practice-related activity.

For example, imagine a nurse in a genito-urinary clinic reading something in *NT* about dying with dignity: an article looking at different cultural beliefs surrounding death. Although working with death is not usually a feature of her working day, the nurse realises that sexuality and sexual taboos are very significant in the location where she works, which has a large population from an Asian background. The nurse realises that despite this, relatively few Asian clients present at her clinic so she investigates further to find out what social and cultural factors might be at work. As a result of her research the nurse is able to establish an outreach network with local community centres, social clubs and places of work where she gives talks and hands out information in a number of languages stressing the need for early investigation and treatment of genito-urinary disease.

All this activity represents activity relevant to meeting PREP requirements and comes from reading the professional press. We hope that the materials in the book will similarly stimulate your personal and professional development.

The Study Hours logo is a registered trade mark of Emap Healthcare Ltd

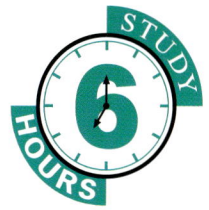

Eating disorders
Knowledge for practice

The term eating disorders covers a wide spectrum of conditions characterised by psychological and behavioural disturbances associated with weight, food and eating (Myers et al, 1993).

The term is often used with reference to two specific conditions: anorexia nervosa (AN) and bulimia nervosa (BN). The relationship between the different types of eating disorder remains unclear.

ANOREXIA NERVOSA AND BULIMIA NERVOSA

There are many misleading stereotypes relating to those who develop AN and BN. The conditions are often portrayed as affecting only young women from higher social classes.

The reality is that in the developed world, both men and women of any age or background can develop these disorders, although it is true that both are far more common in females.

Males account for only one in 10 of those with AN and one in 20 of those with BN. The prevalence of BN is estimated at being between 1–2% of the 16 to 40 age group, whereas AN is found in about 0.5% of this population, rising to 8% in high-risk groups such as models and dancers. Both disorders are related to normal behaviour and concerns; for example up to 90% of women have been on slimming diets and 10% have at some time used vomiting and laxative abuse in an attempt to control their weight (Dolan, 1991).

WHAT IS ANOREXIA NERVOSA?

This term anorexia nervosa is somewhat misleading as 'anorexia' implies loss of appetite. Yet people with this condition have increased appetite because they are starving and experience a constant internal battle between the desire to eat and fear of the consequences of so doing.

Usually, AN takes hold during adolescence. It can persist throughout life and may cause death if not successfully treated. It is known as a psychosomatic disorder, which means that it involves both the body and the mind. It is characterised by a marked loss of weight or failure to gain weight during growth and a fear of being a normal weight for age and height.

People with AN are unable to allow themselves to eat normally as they are terrified of gaining weight. Their relentless pursuit of low weight often gives rise to a dangerous situation, as their behaviour spirals out of control. They may be dramatically underweight and be at considerable physical risk.

People with AN frequently describe a sense of loss of control over their lives, and a feeling of being powerless to change their behaviours.

Despite the situation in which they find themselves, people with AN often appear to have significant reservations at the prospect of engaging in treatment. This ambivalence is central to the condition: individuals are torn between feeling relief when they lose weight and being frightened by what is happening to them. They are often reluctant to seek help and may find themselves coerced into treatment by concerned family and friends. However, to them, attending for treatment implies relinquishing the control and influence they exert over their food and eating.

Usually, patients do not want to be treated for their disorder as it serves to protect them from psychological pain and they feel worse without having it (Crisp and McClelland, 1996). AN always develops as a 'solution' to problems in life. Thus, in some respects, AN can be described as a symptom or physical manifestation of underlying psychological problems.

Diagnosis

Anorexia nervosa has been described for many centuries, and since it was named in 1874 many have struggled to categorise it.

The precise aetiology is much debated, but a combination of genetic, social and intrapersonal factors is thought to be implicated. The diagnostic criteria are shown in Table 1.

In practice, it often happens that patients do not meet all of the criteria and the boundaries of the condition can be unclear.

There are also difficulties establishing a normal weight

Table 1. Diagnostic criteria for anorexia nervosa

- Refusal to maintain body weight over a minimum normal weight for age and height (weight loss leading to body weight 15% below that expected)

- Failure to make expected weight gain during a period of growth, leading to body weight 15% below that expected

- Intense fear of gaining weight or of becoming fat even though underweight

- Disturbance in the way in which the person regards his/her body weight, size, or shape: undue attention to body shape and weight on self-evaluation, or denial of the seriousness of low body weight

- In females absence of at least three consecutive menstrual cycles when they would normally be expected to occur (primary or secondary amenorrhoea) (DSM, 1993).

or an abnormal body image for individuals, as there is a lack of appropriate data on the normal population.

Symptoms of AN

The central symptoms of AN are those common to starvation, together with a preoccupation with body weight and a fear of being a normal weight. Weight loss is achieved initially through restricting calorie intake. This causes a wide range of physical, behavioural and mental state changes, many of which are a direct result of starvation, rather than being particular to AN.

As weight loss increases, muscle and other body tissue is metabolised to provide energy. This occurs more quickly in males and young people, who have less body fat than adult women.

Metabolic rate slows down to conserve energy, and blood supply to the extremities is reduced. Patients feel the cold, suffer rhinitis and develop symptoms similar to Raynaud's syndrome. They may develop lanugo (fine hair) on their bodies to conserve heat, as do premature babies.

Malnutrition can result in anaemia, constipation and vitamin deficiency. Menstruation stops in females (initially as a result of severe carbohydrate restriction) and libido reduces. Dehydration is common in AN, and in severe cases can result in hypokalemia, with impaired cardiac and renal function.

Patients notice that their skin is dry and their hair and nails brittle. Autoimmune function is generally heightened until very low body weight (BMI <13, see Fig 2) is achieved, when it is reduced.

Mentally, patients experience a sense of well-being as they lose weight. At the same time, their thinking becomes more concrete and they become less aware of their feelings. They also become restless and agitated, have difficulty in concentrating and in making simple decisions.

Their starving state generates intense hunger and preoccupation with food and waking hours are spent planning how to eke out their modest allowances: they may dream about food, hoard food, read about food and make it for others. Starvation may be associated with shoplifting and stealing. Patients feel frightened a lot of the time, but are unable to admit this to others. They may also lie about their behaviour for fear that others will interfere.

People with a fear of weight gain may repeatedly weigh themselves, perhaps even several times a day. Despite this they are unable to judge their weight accurately and may perceive themselves as being fat even though underweight. However, many people with anorexia realise that they are thin, but are unable to appreciate the consequences of this.

Socially, patients become increasingly isolated, as their mental state revolves increasingly around food and weight control, and they are unable to cope with social situations, many of which involve eating and drinking. Sometimes they become more studious or more dedicated to their work, which may be commended by others initially, but they can have depression secondary to starvation and sleep is often poor as a result of hunger. These symptoms can easily be confused with those of depressive illness.

Most of the above symptoms are biological responses to starvation and disappear if the patient's nutritional state can be improved. The body appears able to survive even severe malnutrition without long-term adverse consequences.

Other behaviours used to 'control' body weight

Laxative abuse and vomiting are two of the most common methods used in addition to restriction of food intake. Patients often believe that by taking large quantities of laxatives they can prevent calorie absorption after eating. In fact, laxatives work on the large bowel, following digestion, and simply speed up the bowel activity, preventing water and water soluble minerals, such as potassium, from being absorbed from food. This can be life-threatening and also cause permanent damage to the bowel.

Self-induced vomiting is another strategy to prevent calorie absorption following eating. It usually occurs when a person has been unable to eat in a restricted way or has 'broken the rules' he/she has previously set. It is more effective than laxative abuse in preventing calorie absorption, although not completely effective.

Like laxative abuse, it results in dehydration, as well as gastric and oesophageal ulceration, damage to dental enamel, hiatus hernia and gastric reflux. Self-induced vomiting can become automatic and is a very difficult habit to break.

Excessive exercise is used by many people with anorexia to burn up calories; it also helps them to manage their anxiety. It has a moderate effect on energy expenditure, but less than most people imagine, particularly in view of low weight and reduced metabolic rate. Nevertheless, excessive exercise causes additional stress on impaired cardiac function and bone density. Men are particularly likely to use exercise as a means of weight control.

Other strategies for controlling weight are fluid restriction, especially in children, and drug use/abuse — notably diuretics, amphetamines and insulin. Most of these additional behaviours are more risky than simple abstinence and gradual weight loss, and therefore treatment interventions need to be targeted particularly at these.

BULIMIA NERVOSA

Bulimia nervosa is also a psychosomatic disorder but, in contrast to AN, people with BN experience serious loss of control over their appetite and eating. They can eat exceptionally large amounts of food (bulimia literally means 'ox hunger') and then engage in compensatory behaviours to prevent weight gain. While people with AN appear reluctant to be treated for their disorder, those with BN generally wish to be free of it. They often feel too embarrassed and ashamed of their behaviour to tell anyone about it and the condition is often kept secret.

People with BN are usually of normal or near normal body weight. Despite this apparent normality they are pre-occupied with thoughts about food, weight, shopping, cooking, bingeing and finally getting rid of food. People with BN often find that once they start eating they lose control and are not able to limit their intake.

This can lead them to restricting their food intake drastically and eating only when they know they can purge afterwards. In fact, those who develop BN always begin with a period of dietary restriction; the binge eating seems to develop as a (normal) reaction to excessive restriction. The disorder then becomes self-perpetuating as binge-eating is followed by restriction which then leads to further bingeing.

Diagnosis

BN was defined as a distinct condition only in 1979 (Russell, 1979). However, like anorexia nervosa it has probably existed for centuries. The criteria for BN in the *Diagnostic and Statistical Manual of Mental Disorders* (DSM IV) are shown in Table 2.

About 40% of people who develop BN have previously had AN. Occasionally, people swing between the two conditions and binge-eating can sometimes be a feature of AN. BN appears to be a way of regulating and suppressing often disturbing emotions and is associated with very poor self-esteem.

Symptoms of BN

The central symptoms of BN are preoccupation with weight and shape, binge-eating, fear of loss of control of eating and compensatory behaviour to prevent weight gain following bingeing. The person is terrified of losing control of eating and of gaining weight. These fears lead to entrenched patterns of behaviour and a feeling of lack of self-control. Bingeing can become a substitute for emotions.

After bingeing the person describes being exhausted and drained but less troubled by feelings and emotions. A sense of relief is common, although guilt and depression can increase.

Many of the features common to AN are also found in BN, although they are not the result of starvation. Food and weight gain become central to the individual's life, which becomes focused around attempts to control them. Unlike those with AN, people with BN are usually able to conceal their disorder from others, therefore it has less impact on their social functioning. However, this results in their leading a 'double life' which may be outwardly successful but subjectively full of shame, guilt and a profound sense of failure.

Many become extremely depressed about their situation and suicidal thinking and behaviour is not uncommon in this group. The high-risk behaviours found in AN are also present in BN, and menstrual disturbances are common in women, with a correlation between polycystic ovarian syndrome and BN. Often these patients present in fertility clinics, where their eating behaviour is unlikely to be assessed.

TREATMENT FOR EATING DISORDERS

Treatment for eating disorders usually involves a combination of physical and psychological management, reflecting the psychosomatic nature of these disorders. Treatment may be carried out in a variety of settings, with most people remaining in the community during treatment.

People with BN often respond well to a short course of cognitive behavioural treatment aimed at normalising their eating pattern, reducing bingeing and purging behaviour and managing their thoughts and feelings in a more healthy manner. Selective serotonin reuptake inhibitors (SSRIs) such as Prozac and Seroxat appear to be useful for some people in limiting binge eating and improving mood. Counselling and psychotherapy are also useful (Fairburn and Wilson, 1995).

The treatment of AN is more complex and usually more extended than that for BN. This is partly because engagement and the establishment of a therapeutic relationship is more complex.

The life-threatening nature of AN also makes hospital treatment more likely, although most people can be treated out of hospital.

The aims of treatment are to restore normal eating and a healthy weight, while helping the clients discover what their underlying difficulties are and how to manage them in a more healthy way. For those with AN, treatment can be complicated by the fact that when they look more 'nor-

EATING DISORDERS

mal', others are relieved, whereas they themselves feel out of control and are exposed to the difficulties which precipitated the disorder in the first place. If this dilemma is not successfully managed, further weight loss can ensue.

Family therapy has been shown to be very successful in young people with AN (Russell et al, 1997), but otherwise there is no best treatment for the disorder. Treatment usually involves a combination of dietary and weight management, individual and family therapy and occupational therapy.

Cognitive therapy can be useful for some people and motivational work may be necessary in the early stages of treatment. Drug treatment is acknowledged to be unsuitable in AN other than to manage distress or anxiety.

Recovery is possible in both BN and AN, however in a minority of people the conditions become chronic, with consequent increase in health risks and secondary effects on quality of life. It remains unclear why some people recover and others remain ill. Approximately 10% of people with AN will die as a result of their condition, usually from suicide, cardiac arrest or starvation. This gives AN one of the highest death rates of any mental health problem. The proportion who die as a result of BN is unknown.

THINKING POINTS

● What are the factors that influence an individual's recovery from AN? Write down all those you can think of.
● How do attitudes to binge-eating differ between cultures? Read about the attitudes and practices in relation to food and weight of those from non-Western cultures.
● What are the long-term physical, psychological and social consequences for someone of having chronic AN or BN? Compare these with another chronic illness with which you are familiar.

PART TWO

The role of the nurse

The treatment of patients with eating disorders involves both physical and psychological care. Treatment may take place in a variety of settings: in general medical wards, acute psychiatric wards, paediatric wards, adolescent units, specialist eating disorder units, and in community, day and primary care settings. Although many professionals are involved in the care and treatment of these patients, nursing care is generally acknowledged to be of primary importance to this client group (Russell, 1970).

THE THERAPEUTIC RELATIONSHIP

Establishing and maintaining a successful therapeutic relationship is probably the single most important factor in the nursing care of patients with eating disorders. All aspects of the patient's treatment from assessment to evaluation depend on this relationship.

People with eating disorders present in a number of different ways and very few will volunteer details of their difficulties.

This is because they are afraid of people's responses, value judgements and the consequences of revealing information to others. The majority of people with eating disorders are intensely ashamed of their eating behaviour and of their difficulties and are terrified of losing control of these.

The nurse, therefore, has the important job of establishing a safe and trusting relationship within which patients can begin to reveal their difficulties and the extent of their disordered eating.

People with anorexia nervosa (AN), particularly, will be unlikely to volunteer information unless asked directly. This means that the nurse needs to have an understanding of the eating disorder and its associated psychopathology in order to build a relationship.

Open-ended questions can be very difficult for people with eating disorders to answer, since they do not know what the expected or acceptable answer is. As a result, they may say nothing or give an answer which they think is 'right', but which may not be true. This can lead to many misunderstandings in relationships, and the nurse needs to be constantly alert to this possibility.

Key elements of successful therapeutic relationships with people who have eating disorders are:
● Reliability and consistency — keeping appointments, letting the patient know when you are on or off-duty, telling the patient what is going to happen, delivering what has been agreed
● Clarity and structure — establishing a clear programme of care, making decisions and sticking to them (especially when under pressure not to), making expectations explicit
● Honesty — being truthful to the patient at all times is important, even if this is difficult (for example if the patient is under threat of being kept in hospital under a section of the Mental Health Act, or you do not feel able to trust him/her)
● Managing anxiety — do not make management decisions in response to panic about the patient, help family members to manage their anxiety and concern, and look at risky behaviour in context
● Managing boundaries — being wary about sharing your personal information, especially regarding eating and

weight and relationships; planning for discharge or the ending of the relationship, paying attention to the beginning and ending of each therapeutic contact.

These basic principles are important in all settings, from general medical settings to specialist mental health settings.

Nurses have the greatest opportunity to develop therapeutic relationships with these patients, without which treatment will be unsuccessful.

NEEDS OF PATIENTS

People with eating disorders have difficulties in a wide range of areas, which vary from individual to individual. Their needs cross physical and psychological health boundaries and successful nursing care depends on an understanding of the relationship between mind and body and an ability to link the two.

The most common areas of need and difficulty in eating disorders are:
● Weight and dietary management

● Physical and psychological development
● Mood
● Understanding and managing feelings
● Understanding and managing interpersonal relationships
● Self-care and identifying needs and wants
● Self-concept and self-esteem
● Structuring time and leisure activities.

WEIGHT AND DIETARY MANAGEMENT

The area of weight and dietary management is fraught with difficulty for patients with an eating disorder. Many professionals, including nurses, can feel ill-equipped to manage these issues and it is often in this area that major difficulties are encountered in nursing these patients. However, the basic principles underlying weight and dietary management are relatively simple.

Body tissue is largely made up of water. In females, water accounts for up to 80% of body composition; in men the proportion is slightly less. Muscle, bone, fat and

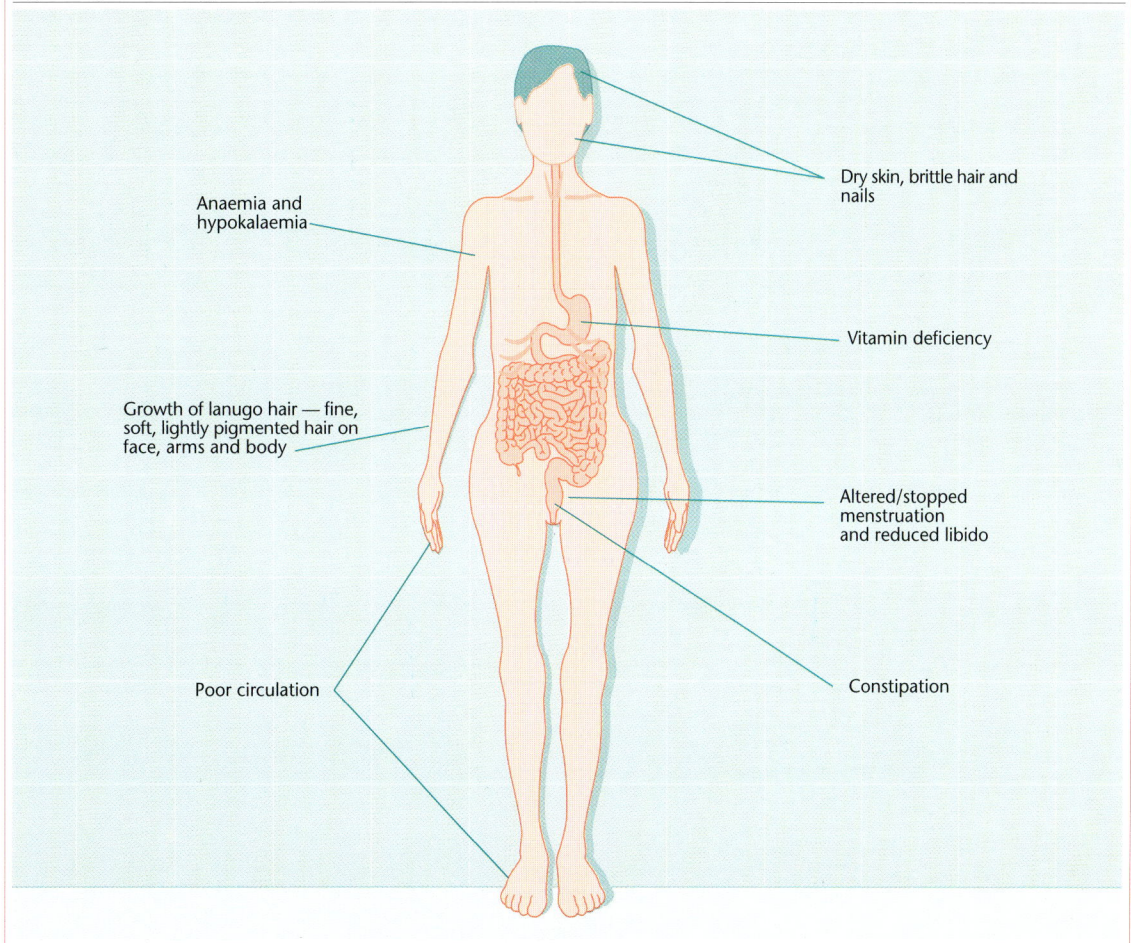

Fig 1. Physical changes resulting from starvation

Dry skin, brittle hair and nails

Anaemia and hypokalaemia

Vitamin deficiency

Growth of lanugo hair — fine, soft, lightly pigmented hair on face, arms and body

Altered/stopped menstruation and reduced libido

Poor circulation

Constipation

connective tissue account for the remainder. This also means that weight is dependent on fluid balance — fluctuations in weight of more than about 1kg per week result from changes in water content.

When the body is normally hydrated, weight stays fairly constant unless there is an imbalance of energy intake versus output.

An imbalance of approximately 3,500kcal will cause a change in weight of approximately 0.5kg. So if people eat 13,500 kcal in a week, but use up only 10,000kcal, their weight will increase by 0.5kg.

The problems that many people with eating disorders have in managing their weight and diet stem in part from their fears about their own weight and partly from a set of mistaken beliefs about weight driven by these fears. The nurse therefore has an important role in educating patients about weight, energy intake, the role of fluid balance, and the real effects of vomiting and laxative abuse.

For example, many patients who believe that laxative abuse causes them to 'lose weight' will seek to stop this when they realise that it has no effect on calorie ingestion and only damages the bowel, causes severe electrolyte imbalance, and dehydrates them.

The issue of weight and weight management can be a problematic issue for nurses, many of whom have their own concerns about weight.

Being weighed in the presence of another person is terrifying for most people with eating disorders. A few 'golden rules' about weighing can make the situation easier for all parties.

● Do not weigh too often, as it is confusing and stressful for patients. Once or twice a week is fine, if possible at the same time of day

● Involve patients in setting a 'target' weight. Clear weight goals and/or bands are very useful and provide safety

● If an anorectic patient is unable to consider a weight goal, a medically safe weight should be chosen (usually BMI 14-15). Setting goals which are too high for patients leads to undue distress and almost certain failure for all

● As far as possible give patients choice when weighing takes place, that is, days and times. It is important to stick to these

● Try and ensure that patients are weighed by someone they know

● Always tell patients their weight unless they ask you not to. Charting weight can be useful as it gives a visual record of what is happening

● Make sure that there is time following weighing for patients to discuss their feelings about their weight if they want to

● Do not expect patients to be open about how they feel. A change in weight which is reassuring for staff is usually the opposite for a patient, and vice-versa

● Give plenty of encouragement without being too pressurising.

In AN, weight gain should be a maximum of 1–2kg/week for in-patients, and 0.5–1kg for those who are outpatients, except in the initial stages when rehydration is occurring. In BN, achieving weight stability is usually the goal.

Dietary management is an equally difficult area. Patients have many fears and beliefs about eating and about the safety or danger of certain foods. In hospital, they will be terrified at the idea of having no control over their food.

In most cases, dietitians will be involved at least at assessment, but the nursing staff are almost always responsible for the ongoing dietary management.

Where possible accommodate patients' beliefs and food preferences, building on 'safe' foods and gradually introducing less safe ones. This is a very important part of relationship-building with patients, and successful management can depend on getting it right. Some useful strategies are:

● As far as possible establish a clear diet plan with details of times, food and fluid intake. Ensure adequate carbohydrate intake, especially where binge eating is a problem

● Keep the plan simple. It is important that patients receive what has been planned, otherwise they will be unable to trust you. Cheese sandwiches for lunch every day are 'safer' than a varied diet which cannot be guaranteed

● Include some foods with which the patient feels safe, even if they are foods low in calories

● If possible, allow patients to eat in their room or somewhere private, unless they request otherwise

● Do not encourage the eating of extra food or eating at times which have not been agreed; this is frightening for patients

● People with eating disorders may find it very difficult to make decisions about food, especially under stress; expecting them to do this under pressure is not reasonable

● If patients are not to be given choice about their food and fluid intake or cannot make a decision, staff need to make clear decisions on their behalf and carry them out as soon as possible; for example, in the event of nasogastric feeding

● Keeping a food diary or written record of food and fluid consumed can help patients to feel safer and may be used to manage anxiety

● Many people welcome support after eating, when they feel very panicky and may be tempted to induce vomiting, exercise or binge. Often a distracting activity can be helpful until the anxiety subsides.

DEVELOPMENT

Most people develop eating disorders during adolescence. Those who develop them later have usually had difficulties during adolescent and young adult development. Eating disorders involve both physical and psychological development: bodily changes (including the onset of menstruation in females), cognitive and emotional changes, changes in social roles and functioning. Fig 1 illustrates some of the physical changes which result from starvation.

The normal tasks of adolescence in our society are to achieve physical and psychological maturity, establish sexual identity, separate from families of origin, and to achieve independence, supported by a range of new relationships.

Nurses have a key educational and supportive role for patients, who often have little idea of what is 'normal' and are frightened of internal and external change and growth.

Nurses can also act as important role models for patients, drawing on their own experiences.

MOOD AND MANAGING EMOTIONS

People with eating disorders often have severe difficulty managing their moods and emotions. Many of them are alexythymic, which means that they have an inability to put feelings into words.

They are often out of touch with their feelings and unable to communicate them other than through their body or through their disordered eating.

This deficiency in handling emotions is often at odds with their intellectual ability, so they give the impression of coping well, when in fact they are unable to deal with even straightforward issues in daily life on an emotional level.

They have a great fear of experiencing any emotion, believing it will overwhelm them, and so do their best to prevent themselves feeling anything or to get rid of any feelings they do have.

Nurses who work closely with these patients can often find themselves experiencing the emotion 'on behalf of' the patient.

This can lead to conflicts between staff members which reflect the emotional conflicts being experienced by patients.

The role of the nurse is to manage and contain feelings which patients are unable to bear, very much in the same way as a parent may do for a child, so that patients can learn to tolerate and manage the feelings for themselves. The nurse can also help them to make sense of their feelings.

Patients with eating disorders also suffer disturbances of mood, particularly during treatment. It is common, for example, for people with AN to experience depression as their weight becomes more normal.

Usually this is a positive sign — the patient may have plenty of things to be depressed about — but the nurse needs to monitor each patient's mental state, as sometimes the depression can be severe and require treatment.

Patients can also resort to self-harming behaviours as a way of managing their feelings, and in extreme cases can attempt suicide.

These problems need to be taken seriously, as they are signs of an inability to cope with feelings.

INTERPERSONAL RELATIONSHIPS

People with eating disorders often have great difficulty in managing relationships of all kinds. They are generally insecure and depend on the approval of others, as they have little sense of self worth or value.

They may constantly try to please others or to work out what others want or expect from them. They are particularly afraid of managing dependent relationships, feeling that their needs are too great or that they will be rejected by others.

Relationships with others are fraught with fear, and patients may present as withdrawn, hostile, compliant, angry or distressed as a way of trying to manage their relationships with others.

For nurses managing these relationships requires skill and patience and a willingness to 'read between the lines'. Consistency on the part of staff, particularly nurses, is an especially important part of the work.

SELF-CARE AND SELF-ESTEEM

Because of the deficit in self-esteem which is common to people with eating disorders, they may have difficulty managing aspects of their self-care which others take for granted.

Often these deficits are in the areas of food and eating, but they can also extend to difficulties with self-harming behaviours, lacking adequate clothing and heating for themselves, an inability to spend money on themselves appropriately, depriving themselves of rest and sleep, overworking, and so on.

Cognitive and behavioural strategies are useful in managing many of these difficulties and often practical help is needed — perhaps with shopping, budgeting, structuring time and planning leisure activities.

Self-harming behaviours, such as cutting, overdosing, drug and alcohol abuse are signs of very severe psychological difficulties and require careful management, as the resolution of one problem may lead the person to develop another.

As with the eating disorder symptoms, these behaviours represent ways of coping and need to be understood as such.

SUMMARY

The role of the nurse in the treatment of eating disorders requires a wide range of skills and confidence in managing high levels of anxiety.

For many patients, the nurse is the key professional involved in their care and is in a position to offer significant treatment and support to individuals who suffer these distressing problems.

THINKING POINTS

● What are your beliefs and expectations about people who have eating disorders? List these and think how they may affect your approach to building therapeutic relationships with such patients.
● What are your feelings and attitudes about your own weight and that of friends and colleagues? Consider how weight affects perceptions and expectations of others.
● How does your eating pattern change according to how you feel and what you are doing?

Keep a diary for a week recording your eating behaviour, mood and general activity.
Look for patterns of behaviour.
● What is 'normal' adolescent development? Write down the key experiences and memories from your own adolescence. Share these with a friend or colleague and compare notes.
● Where does self-esteem come from and how is it reflected in life? Think of two people you know well, write down your impressions of their self-esteem and how you made this judgement about them.

PART THREE

Professional issues

The treatment of people with eating disorders brings up many issues for consideration in relation to nursing practice. The nurse-patient relationship in eating disorders can be complex, and the notions of power and control are central features of it. People with anorexia nervosa (AN), in particular, are often perceived as difficult to nurse.

Ethical issues over the patient's right to refuse treatment and professionals' responsibilities to treat the patient can be the cause of apparent conflicts of interest between patients and professionals.

These disorders occur predominantly in females, and in recent years feminist and female understandings of these problems have radically reshaped the way the disorders are understood and approached.

The views of patients about their treatment and their difficulties have until recently been almost entirely ignored by professionals. This, too, is starting to change, resulting in more individualised and less rigid approaches to treatment for eating disorders.

POWER AND CONTROL

The issues of power and control are central features of eating disorders. Patients perceive themselves as lacking in self-control and self-discipline and as powerless to effect change in their problematic eating behaviour or in their lives in general. In contrast to this, the experience of those around the patient may be that the disorder makes them very controlling and powerful.

Treatment approaches to these disorders have traditionally focused on taking control of problematic behaviours; although this was and is helpful to many, it can lead to considerable conflict between staff and patients, particularly for nurses. In addition, patients' fear and mistrust of professionals and treatment, juxtaposed with their desire for approval, can lead to profound misunderstandings between staff and patients, with patients being perceived as deceitful and manipulative and staff becoming involved in increasingly invasive and restrictive attempts to enforce patients' co-operation with treatment.

Each person's ability to take control over their eating disorder will vary according to the severity of the disorder, his/her underlying problems and the nature of the help given.

At one end of the spectrum, a person may be able to manage with minimal or no help from professionals, whereas another may end up being detained under a section of the Mental Health Act as a life-saving measure or perhaps even be denied treatment because of being unable to 'abide by the rules' which the professionals have set.

CHOICE AND EMPOWERMENT

Many people with eating disorders are able to manage their lives independently and hold down jobs, cope with their studies or run a household. However, when people are unable to keep their weight and/or eating within socially acceptable limits, assumptions are often made about their ability to regulate and control other areas of their life. In this way, control and choice can often be taken away by professionals 'who know best'.

Empowering patients to make their own choices about their treatment is something that, arguably, nurses are best placed to do (Pullen, 1995). Nurses have a privileged position in this respect because of the amount of contact they have with patients and the holistic nature of their training.

Exercising this choice when faced with someone with AN who is a dangerously low weight or someone with bulimia nervosa (BN) whose eating appears dangerously

EATING DISORDERS

out of control requires skill and experience and an awareness of professional and personal competence.

In a study carried out on behalf of the Eating Disorders Association, 50% of patients who had been detained under the Mental Health Act because of their eating disorder were glad that professionals had taken this decision (Newton et al, 1993). However, the feelings of the other 50% are unclear.

Helping patients to make choices in situations such as these requires that nurses acknowledge their power and use it to help patients.

For example, offering clear and unbiased information about the situation, outlining the short- and long-term risks and the treatment options, making clinical records and other clinical information available, using clear and straightforward language, clarifying patients' understanding, and actively seeking their views at all stages of care delivery.

In circumstances where the nurse has to make or contribute to the making of a decision on behalf of a patient, it is important to be open about this, explain the rationale and the consequences of the decision to the patient. Learning to manage one's own anxiety in these situations is essential for nurses. Knowledge and experience can empower nurses to offer choices to patients, even in high-risk situations.

ACCESS TO TREATMENT

Access to appropriate treatment for people with eating disorders remains problematic (Hogg, 1994). There are few specialist NHS services, most of them are for adults, and these are spread unevenly across the UK. Many private providers now offer treatment for eating disorders, having perceived 'a gap in the market'.

The internal market in the NHS further increased difficulties, with some purchasers refusing to pay for specialist treatment or permitting treatment only with certain providers.

Some people, especially young people, can end up being treated for months in units many miles from where they live.

Local services are being set up in many areas, but staff lack the support and expertise to work in this area, particularly as there is a serious lack of specialist training and supervision available to professionals.

Patients complain that they are too often seen by professionals who know nothing about their problems and who do not understand them. Inappropriate treatment can be very damaging for patients and so the more that nurses can learn about these problems, the more they will be able to help patients in their care.

INDIVIDUALISED CARE AND TREATMENT

Specialist treatment for eating disorders in recent decades has normally followed a standardised approach, whereby patients are admitted to a treatment programme for their

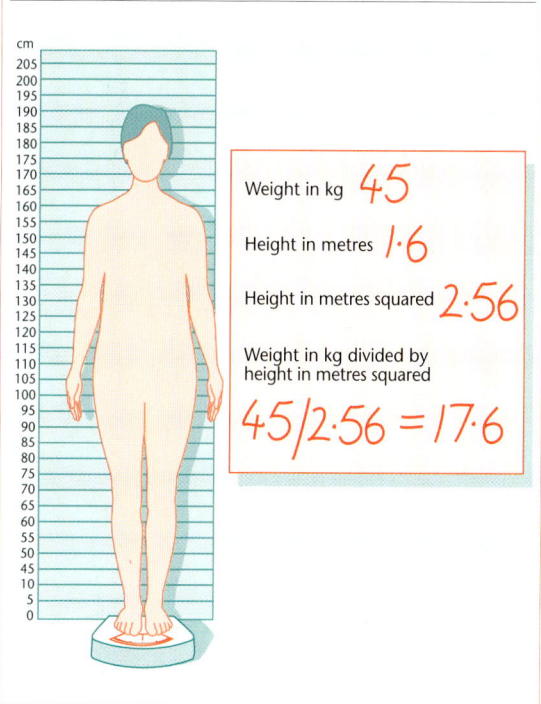

Fig 2. The calculation of body mass index

Weight in kg *45*

Height in metres *1·6*

Height in metres squared *2·56*

Weight in kg divided by height in metres squared

$$45/2·56 = 17·6$$

particular disorder and are expected to achieve a number of milestones during their treatment. The majority of such treatment programmes are aimed at recovery from the eating disorder.

Many people with eating disorders complain that these programmes do not respect their individuality, are inflexible and offer them no choice.

Because specialist treatment options remain limited in this country, many patients feel they have no choice but to accept a regime they do not feel is suitable for them, often because they are desperate for help. Nurses in such units may have to struggle to provide individualised care within the limitations of the treatment programmes.

However, treatment for eating disorders is gradually becoming more flexible and individualised, although much remains to be done in this area, especially for those people who have long-term or chronic difficulties and who cannot aim for recovery in the short term. Many of these people feel that they have failed the treatment programmes, rather than that the programmes are unsuited to their needs.

A nursing approach based on an holistic model, such as that used at Annex (Halek et al, 1995), allows each individual's needs to be assessed and managed according to the severity of their problems, their expressed wishes and their strengths and weaknesses.

Similarly, the women's movement, with its alternative ways of understanding and living with eating disorders, has pioneered more tolerant and compassionate approaches to these disorders (Lawrence, 1987).

MEN WITH EATING DISORDERS

Eating disorders primarily affect females. However, about 5% of people with eating disorders are male and the disorders present in very similar ways in males and females. In children about 50% of those affected are boys, but prevalence changes dramatically after puberty. Males with eating disorders face particular problems in treatment, because the area is so female dominated.

Available literature, therapeutic interventions and environments are overwhelmingly biased towards females and because of this, treatment for males can be isolating and alienating. It is important for nurses to be aware of this and to try to provide male patients with gender-appropriate interventions and literature where possible.

COMPLEMENTARY THERAPIES

Many people with eating disorders report that they find complementary and non-verbal therapies helpful. Those that seem particularly useful are dance and movement therapies, art and music therapies, body image work, physical therapies such as massage and reflexology, and aromatherapy. Some people who do not respond to more conventional medically-based treatments may benefit from a complementary therapy approach. Because of the physical complications of these disorders and the difficulties in managing boundaries, it is important that these therapies are carried out in conjunction with expert supervision.

USER INVOLVEMENT

Until very recently, user involvement was almost unheard of in the field of eating disorders, despite the existence of a national self-help organisation (the Eating Disorders Association — EDA), and a considerable user movement in other areas of mental health (Mind, Survivors Speak Out).

Over the past five years, this picture has gradually begun to alter. In 1994, EDA published service specifications for providers and purchasers of eating disorder services and for those working in primary care settings (Hogg, 1994).

Research has been published in association with the Royal College of Psychiatrists about users' views of treatment (Newton et al, 1993) and gradually some services are beginning to incorporate users' views into their service development and to encourage service-users to participate more actively in their treatment.

However, there is a long way to go in this area, and there is still a belief that people with eating disorders are not capable of making sensible decisions and choices about their treatment.

The problems often arise because the choices that patients might make are not those that professionals would make. Many people with eating disorders never approach services for help, or opt out at the earliest possible opportunity because of this. There is a real challenge for nurses working in this field to accommodate the wishes of patients as far as possible and to act as advocates for patients in situations of conflict. This requires nurses to examine their own reasons for their preferences and choices about a person's treatment and to be honest about them.

ACUTE VERSUS CHRONIC MODELS OF CARE

Much treatment available in the field of eating disorders is based on acute models of care, whereby a disorder is diagnosed and a treatment method chosen which is designed to 'cure' it. However, as eating disorders represent people's attempts to cope with life, patients do not respond so easily to this approach. It is not possible for people to be 'cured' unless they are able to develop other ways of coping with life. This can be extremely difficult or even impossible for some people to achieve.

The average length of a treatment episode for someone with BN is two years and for someone with AN three years. However, about 10% of people will experience a severe and chronic form of their disorder, which may persist throughout life. Long-term studies of AN show that recovery is possible even after more than 20 years with the disorder (Theander, 1983).

RESEARCH, EDUCATION AND DEVELOPMENT

Research into eating disorders remains an important and thriving area, particularly as so much remains unknown or inconclusive. Current areas of research interest are aetiology of the disorders, long-term effects on health (osteoporosis, fertility), outcome of treatment, the search for optimum treatments and the use of medication in BN. It is very difficult to secure funding for research into eating disorders, as so little of the treatment is medical, and pharmacology, in particular, plays a very small part in treatment.

Special interest groups exist within the Royal College of Psychiatrists, the Royal College of Nursing and the British Dietetic Association for professionals working with or interested in eating disorders. These are important forums for the exchange of knowledge and information between professionals.

Education and training in the field of eating disorders are difficult to come by. Most nurses (and others) specialising in this field have learnt their skills by working in specialist units, for example, on an apprenticeship model.

There is a course for nurses at the University of Birmingham, which offers an eating disorder pathway within an MSc in Health Studies. Other courses are being developed at Colchester (which is offering an ENB course) and in London. A number of study days and workshops are offered by specialist units around the country and it is worth keeping an eye out for them.

The Women's Therapy Centre in London also offers training in this area, but their courses are mainly open only to women. Major conferences are held in the UK and elsewhere, and provide the main way for professionals to keep up to date with developments in the field. There are also a number of professional journals published, notably the *International Journal of Eating Disorders* and *European Eating Disorder Review*, which can be obtained through libraries, or in the case of the latter by professional membership of EDA.

THINKING POINTS

● The UKCC's *Code of Professional Conduct* states that the nurse should 'always act in such a manner as to promote and safeguard the interests and wellbeing of clients and patients'. What do you think the patients might see as their interests when they experience eating disorders? Compare these with the interests of professionals who might be involved.

● What is recovery? Who decides if a person has recovered? Think about the ways in which you cope with your life; how many of these are 'healthy' or 'unhealthy'?

REFERENCES

Crisp, A. H., McClelland, L. (1996) *Anorexia Nervosa: Guidelines for Assessment and Treatment in Primary and Secondary Care*. London: Lawrence Erlbaum.

Dolan, B. (1991) *Why Women? Gender Issues and Eating Disorders*. London: European Council on Eating Disorders, 1991.

Fairburn, C.G., Wilson, G.T. (eds) (1995) *Binge Eating: Nature, Assessment and Treatment*. New York: Guilford Press.

Halek, C. et al (1995) Weight on their minds. *Nursing Times*; 91: 48, 42–43.

Hogg, C. (1994) *Eating Disorders: A Guide to Purchasing and Providing Services*. Norwich: Eating Disorders Association.

Lawrence, M. (1987) *Fed Up and Hungry: Women, Oppression and Food*. London: The Women's Press.

Myers, S. et al (1993) *A General Practitioner's Guide to Eating Disorders*. London: Institute of Psychiatry.

Diagnostic and Statistical Manual of Mental Disorders (DSM IV) (1993) Washington DC: American Psychiatric Association.

Newton, T. et al (1993) Treatment for eating disorders in the United Kingdom. Part II. Experiences of treatment: A survey of members of the Eating Disorders Association. *Eating Disorders Review*; 1: 2, 4–9.

Pullen, F. (1995) Advocacy: a specialist practitioner role. *British Journal of Nursing*; 4: 5.

Russell, G.F.M. (1979) Bulimia nervosa. An ominous variant of anorexia nervosa. *Psychological Medicine*; 9: 429–48.

Russell, G.F.M. et al (1987) An evaluation of family therapy in anorexia nervosa and bulimia nervosa. *Archives of General Psychiatry* 1987; 44: 1047–1056.

Russell, G.F.M. (1970) Anorexia nervosa: its identity as an illness and its treatment. In: Price, J.H. (ed.) *Modern Trends in Psychological Medicine*; 2: 131–164. New York: Appleton-Century-Crofts.

Theander, S. (1983) Research on outcome and prognosis of anorexia nervosa and some results from the Swedish long-term study. *International Journal of Eating Disorders*; 2: 167–174.

FURTHER READING

Crisp, A.H. (1996) *Anorexia Nervosa: Let Me Be*. London: Lawrence Erlbaum Associates.

Duker, M., Slade, R. (1988) *Anorexia Nervosa and Bulimia: How to Help*. Milton Keynes: Open University Press.

Fairburn, C.G., Wilson, G.T. (eds) (1993) *Binge Eating: Nature, Assessment, Treatment*. London: Guilford Press.

Szmukler, G. et al (eds) (1995) *Handbook of Eating Disorders: Theory, Treatment and Research*. London: Wiley.

Useful contacts

Eating Disorders Association
Wensum House
Prince of Wales Road
Norwich,
Norfolk.
Helpline: 01603 621414 (9am-6.30pm Mon-Fri)
Youth helpline (18 and under): 01603 765050
Administration: 01603 619090

The Eating Disorders Association is a national charity offering support and information to people with eating disorders and their families. It produces useful information leaflets, gives information about treatment facilities nationwide and runs a network of self-help groups across the country. It also offers confidential telephone helplines for adults and young people and publishes newsletters. The Association offers professional membership to people working within the field, which includes a subscription to the *European Eating Disorder Review*.

Overeaters Anonymous
PO Box 19, Stretford, Manchester M32 9EB
01426 984674 (information about local groups)

Overeaters Anonymous offers confidential self-help for compulsive eaters run on a 12-step programme similar to Alcoholics Anonymous. A particular characteristic of this organisation is the high level of support offered to people trying to overcome their disorder. The approach is more suitable for people with BN and associated problems than those with AN.

RCN Eating Disorders Special Interest Group
c/o Beverley Murphy
Annex NDU
Harewood House
Springfield Hospital
London SW17 7DJ

Meetings are held every 2–3 months in London

Eating disorders
Assessment

When you have read the unit and completed any further reading, you can use the questions below to test your understanding of the topic. Answers can be found on the next page.

1 Eating disorders are:
- 1 Slimming diseases
- 2 Psychosomatic disorders
- 3 Behavioural problems
- 4 Physical illnesses

2 The central feature of anorexia nervosa is:
- 1 Dieting
- 2 Excessive exercise
- 3 Vomiting
- 4 A fear of being a normal weight

3 Bulimia nervosa is characterised by:
- 1 Episodes of binge eating which are out of control
- 2 Vomiting after normal meals
- 3 Excessive exercise
- 4 Being a normal weight

4 Which of these is a feature of anorexia nervosa but not of bulimia nervosa:
- 1 Being or wishing to be markedly underweight
- 2 Restricting calorie intake
- 3 Abusing laxatives
- 4 Concern about weight and shape

5 The most important aspect of nursing care for people with eating disorders is:
- 1 Maintaining regular food intake
- 2 Establishing a therapeutic relationship
- 3 Controlling the patient's behaviour
- 4 Counselling

6 Which of these causes body weight to fluctuate excessively:
- 1 Eating high calorie food
- 2 Strict dieting
- 3 Excessive exercise
- 4 Dehydration

7 Which of these behaviours presents the greatest short-term risk to a patient's physical health:
- 1 Losing weight
- 2 Exercising
- 3 Laxative abuse
- 4 Restricting calorie intake

8 Any increase in a patient's weight is likely to be accompanied by a corresponding increase in:
- 1 Distress
- 2 Compliance
- 3 Height
- 4 Fluid intake

9 Which of these factors is common to all people with eating disorders:
- 1 Malnutrition
- 2 Poor self-esteem
- 3 Problems in the family
- 4 Lack of education

10 The proportion of men who suffer from eating disorders is:
- 1 Approximately 5% of the general population
- 2 50% of those with eating disorders
- 3 Between 5% and 10% of those with eating disorders
- 4 Unknown

11 Which of these is a central feature of the nurse-patient relationship in eating disorders:
- 1 Manipulative behaviour
- 2 Power and control
- 3 User empowerment
- 4 Powerlessness

12 Eating disorders are an attempt to cope with:
- 1 Being overweight
- 2 Lack of self-control
- 3 Emotional difficulties
- 4 Adolescence

13 Which of these groups of people is most at risk of developing an eating disorder?

1	Middle class females
2	Adolescent females
3	Females under the age of 40
4	Pre-pubertal males

14 Family therapy is a useful treatment in eating disorders for:

1	Young people aged 18 and under
2	People with a long history of the disorder
3	Mothers with young children
4	People with anorexia nervosa

15 Eating disorders mainly occur in the populations of:

1	Western cultures
2	Western and Asian cultures
3	Developed cultures
4	All cultures

16 Eating disorders can result in death in:

1	40–50% of young people under 18
2	10–20% of those with eating disorders
3	10–20% of those with anorexia nervosa
4	5% of those with bulimia nervosa

ANSWERS

Eating disorders

1: Eating disorders are:
1) Psychosomatic disorders

2: The central feature of anorexia nervosa is:
4) A fear of being normal weight

3: Bulimia nervosa is characterised by:
1) Episodes of binge eating that are out of control

4: Which of these is a feature of anorexia nervosa but not of bulimia nervosa:
2) Restricting calorie intake

5: The most important aspect of nursing care for people with eating disorders is:
2) Establishing a therapeutic relationship

6: Which of these causes body weight to fluctuate excessively:
4) Dehydration

7: Which of these behaviours presents the greatest short-term risk to a patient's physical health:
4) Restricting calorie intake

8: Any increase in a patient's weight is likely to be accompanied by a corresponding increase in:
1) Distress

9: Which of these factors is common to all people with eating disorders:
2) Poor self-esteem

10: The proportion of men who suffer from eating disorders is:
3) Between 5% and 10% of those with eating disorders

11: Which of these is a central feature of the nurse-patient relationship in eating disorders:
2) Power and control

12: Eating disorders are an attempt to cope with:
3) Emotional difficulties

13: Which of these groups of people is most at risk of developing an eating disorder?
3) Females under the age of 40

14: Family therapy is a useful treatment in eating disorders for:
1) Young people aged 18 and under

15: Eating disorders mainly occur in the populations of:
1) Western cultures

16: Eating disorders can result in death in:
3) 10–20% of those with anorexia nervosa

11 Clorazil is:

- [ ] 1 Another name for chlorpromazine
- [ ] 2 A new drug that is effective in reducing the side-effects of chlorpromazine
- [ ] 3 A depot medication
- [ ] 4 A psychotropic drug often effective with treatment-resistant psychosis

12 Under the new Supervised Discharge legislation, community mental health nurses have:

- [ ] 1 Responsibility for identifying those people at risk to themselves or others
- [ ] 2 Responsibility for ensuring that prescribed medication is given to people in the community
- [ ] 3 Powers to convey people on Supervised Discharge orders to a place of treatment
- [ ] 4 Powers to place a patient on a section of the Mental Health Act

13 Standardised mortality rates in schizophrenia are:

- [ ] 1 The same as the rest of the population
- [ ] 2 1.5 times those of the rest of the population
- [ ] 3 2.5 times those of the rest of the population
- [ ] 4 3.5 times those of the rest of the population

14 Of the 50% of acute admission to psychiatric wards accounted for by schizophrenia, what proportion stay for more than 6 months?:

- [ ] 1 20%
- [ ] 2 40%
- [ ] 3 60%
- [ ] 4 80%

ANSWERS

Schizophrenia

1: Schizophrenia is most accurately defined as:
3) A diagnosis given to people with thought disorder, auditory hallucinations and delusions

2: The first rank symptoms of schizophrenia were defined by:
4) Schneider

3: Schizophrenia is caused by:
1) A number of interacting factors which lead to vulnerability in the presence of stressor

4: The outcome of schizophrenia is most accurately described by which of the following statements?
4) It is variable: about 30% of people recover completely, 15% have serious disability

5: In relation to the epidemiology of schizophrenia which of the following statements is not true?
3) The incidence of schizophrenia is increasing

6: In relation to informal carers, which of the following statements is not true?
3) People with schizophrenia are more likely to relapse if cared for by family members

7: The role of key worker under the CPA involves which additional skills?
4) Liaison and communication

8: The CPA is best described as:
2) A framework for ensuring assessment, care and planning review

9: The central aim of working with people who have schizophrenia is:
1) Utilising a range of skills and support to enable clients to live their lives as they wish

10: In 1993, the care and treatment costs of people with schizophrenia was estimated to be:
1) £2.6bn

11: Clorazil is:
4) A psychotropic drug often effective with treatment-resistant psychosis

12: Under the new Supervised Discharge legislation, community mental health nurses have:
3) Powers to convey people on Supervised Discharge orders to a place of treatment

13: Standardised mortality rates in schizophrenia are:
3) 2.5 times those of the rest of the population

14: Of the 50% of acute admission to psychiatric wards accounted for by schizophrenia, what proportion stay for more than 6 months?:
3) 60%

Depression in primary care
Knowledge for practice

Relatively few people with depression are referred to specialists and most of them are cared for in primary care settings. It is therefore community nurses who will most frequently encounter patients with depression, not community psychiatric nurses. Nurses in general hospital wards, hospice and residential homes will also see patients with depression and related conditions (Fig 1).

Mental health problems frequently co-exist with physical health problems. People are whole beings; there is no split between mind and body. In nursing terms it makes no sense to care for people's physical needs and ignore their mental health.

WHAT IS DEPRESSION?

Depression, alongside anxiety conditions, is one of a group of psychiatric illnesses known as affective or neurotic disorders. These are disorders of mood, as distinct from psychoses such as schizophrenia, which are disorders of thought. The boundary between the two is not necessarily clear, and some illnesses may have features of both types, particularly if severe. In addition, patients with schizophrenia and organic brain conditions, such as dementia, may also have concurrent depression.

The central feature of depression is a lowering of mood, but for a medical diagnosis of depression to be made, other symptoms must be present (Fig 2). Major depression consists of lowered mood, loss of interest and pleasure,

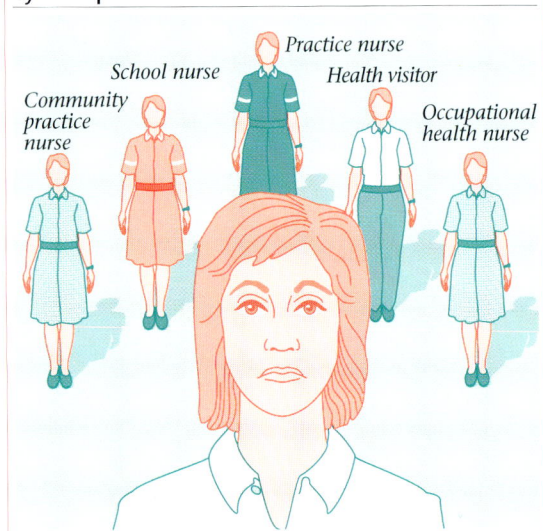

Fig 1. Most depressed people are seen by non-specialist staff

Community practice nurse
School nurse
Practice nurse
Health visitor
Occupational health nurse

plus four or more of the following: feelings of worthlessness or guilt, impaired concentration, loss of energy and fatigue, suicidal thoughts, loss (or increase) of appetite and weight, sleep disturbances (too much or too little), and either slowing down or being agitated.

These symptoms should have been present for a minimum of two weeks and there should be no evidence of primary, underlying disorder (Paykel and Priest, 1992). It is known as unipolar depression to distinguish it from bipolar, or manic, depression, which is characterised by extreme mood swings from severe depressive episodes to high elation or mania. Dysthymia is a lifelong mild fluctuating depression, which may sometimes be exacerbated by more severe acute episodes.

PREVALENCE

A study by the Office of Population Censuses and Surveys showed that about one in seven adults had some form of disturbance of mood in the week prior to interview (Meltzer at al, 1992).

It alos showed that among homeless people the prevalence is about two and a half times that level. The most prevalent disorder among adults was a mixed anxiety and depression syndrome. Women were significantly more likely to experience these problems than men, and the most common symptoms were fatigue, sleep problems, irritability and worry.

There have been many attempts to explain the gender difference in the prevalence of depression. Women may be more able to express feelings than men and are therefore more likely to be diagnosed as depressed. Feminists believe it is related to a power imbalance between female patient and male doctor, and to stereotypical ideas about what constitutes a mentally healthy woman. Others have suggested it is owing to the social pressures on women to bring up a family and have a career. Although rates of affective disorders of all types are highest in divorced people, married men appear to have much lower rates than married women.

Major depression accounts for about 5% of consultations in general practice with a further 5% having symptoms just below this level. Another 10% of patients consulting their GP will have milder illnesses. In about half of these people, the depression may be missed. Clinical studies comparing symptom levels in depression and anxiety of psychiatric hospital patients with those attending their GP surgery have revealed few differences. Moreover, most people who kill themselves have some form of psychiatric disorder, usually depression, and up to two thirds will have consulted their GP in the month prior to the attempt (Department of Health, 1994).

Depression occurs across all ethnic groups, but cultural differences influence the social meaning of mental illnesses and the ways in which people seek help. Communication difficulties and lack of cultural awareness on the part of health professionals may exacerbate the problem of recognition within ethnic groups. Depression also occurs across the age range. It becomes more common with increasing age, but children are not immune. It is possible that 10–20% of children may need help at some time for a mental health disorder. Estimates of the prevalence of depression in children vary and it is necessary to consider psychological disturbances in terms of the individual child's stage of development. For example, whereas an adolescent may react to adverse events by becoming depressed, a younger child may exhibit behavioural difficulties (Armstrong and Tufnell, 1996).

Among older people, community studies have estimated a prevalence of around 15%, although among those attending their GP, rates might be double this. High rates of depression have also been noted in people in residential and care homes. Although depression in older people is strongly associated with physical illness and disability, depression is not a natural consequence of getting old (Katona et al, 1995).

Depression is also common in the postnatal period with around 10–15% of mothers affected. It is important to distinguish postnatal depression from the transient 'baby blues', which affect many more women around the third or fourth postpartum day, and from puerperal psychosis, which affects about one or two women per 1000 and has a dramatic, sudden and early onset (Cox and Holden, 1994).

CAUSES OF DEPRESSION

Psychological, biological and social factors are all implicated in the development of depressive illnesses but no single model is capable of explaining all depression.

Ideas of loss are central to psychological explanations but not all loss, for example bereavement, causes depression. Psychoanalytic theory suggests that the loss that does is of a kind that threatens self-esteem. There also seems to be a role for 'learned helplessness', in which childhood experiences are said to be the origins of a learned sense of being a loser.

The tendency of many depressed patients to view themselves, the world and the future in a negative light may also be important and is the basis of the cognitive theory of depression and the cognitive-behavioural approach to treatment (Delgado et al, 1992).

Biological research has looked at the role played by heredity. Depression, especially manic depression, runs in families. Increasing knowledge about the way antidepressants work has led to theories about the role of brain neurotransmitters, especially serotonin. Disturbances of neurotransmitter systems can cause disturbances of sleep, appetite, motivation and pleasure, all of which may be symptoms of depression. However, it is not always clear whether neurochemical changes cause depression or are caused by it (Royal College of Psychiatrists, 1995).

Major life events and difficulties on their own are not sufficient to cause depression. It may be the meaning that these events have for the person rather than the events themselves that determine whether or not he or she becomes depressed. The relationship between depression and poverty and relationship problems, and the role of emotional, physical and sexual abuse in the development of depressive illnesses in women have been studied (RCP, 1995). Poor personal relationships also contribute to depression in men.

It seems most helpful to consider the aetiology of depression in terms of three sets of factors, predisposing factors, which increase vulnerability or make it likely that the person will develop the illness in the future, precipitating factors, which trigger the illness, and maintaining factors, which prevent the person from recovering (Jenkins et al, 1992). Each factor has biological, social and psychological components, which are summarised in Table 1.

TREATMENT

There are a variety of effective treatments available for depression and no single treatment will suit all patients. A combination of drug therapy and a psychological approach is likely to be most beneficial, but people with severe depression may require medication to lift mood and improve motivation before commencing a 'talking' treatment. It may be helpful to think of treatment options in terms of 'pills for symptoms, talk for problems'.

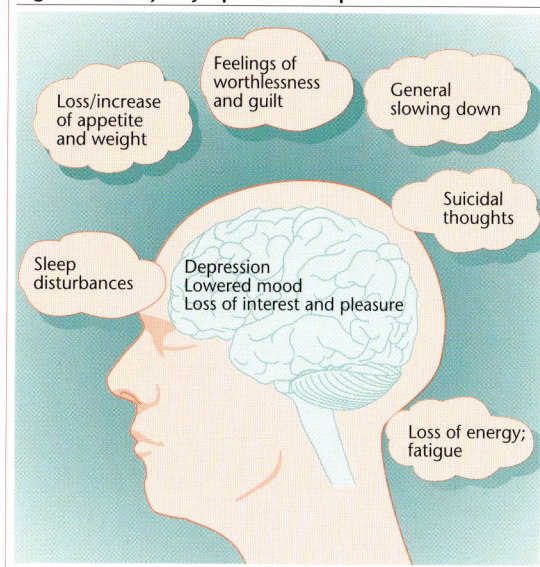

Fig 2. The major symptoms of depression

Loss/increase of appetite and weight

Feelings of worthlessness and guilt

General slowing down

Suicidal thoughts

Sleep disturbances

Depression
Lowered mood
Loss of interest and pleasure

Loss of energy; fatigue

Drug treatment

Patients whose illness reaches the criteria for major depression, including mixed anxiety/depression states, will usually respond to antidepressant treatment whether or not the illness seems understandable. Severe depression feels bad regardless of any supposed cause. Antidepressant drugs have been shown to be effective in moderate to severe depression if given in therapeutic dose for an adequate length of time, and they are not addictive. Antidepressants need to be continued for a minimum of four to six months after the patient begins to feel better and, where the illness is recurrent, lifelong drug treatment may be prescribed.

The tricyclic antidepressants, such as amitriptyline and dothiepin, have been available for many years and are relatively cheap. However, their anticholinergic side-effects are often unpleasant and normally appear before the patient feels any benefit. These drugs are highly toxic in overdose and may be used in suicide attempts. The most significant disadvantage with the tricyclic antidepressants is that they are frequently prescribed at what most experts agree are subtherapeutic doses (Donoghue and Tylee, 1996) and patients do not continue to take their drugs for long enough. Most drugs in this group also have a sedative effect and, whereas this may be helpful for people who have difficulty sleeping, it may increase the risk of accidents, especially in older people.

The selective serotonin re-uptake inhibitors (SSRIs) such as sertraline and fluoxetine have a different side-effect profile and are said to be better tolerated than the tricyclics, but they are also significantly more expensive. An important advantage is that they are less easy to prescribe in low dose. There are also a number of other new antidepressants which act on the noradrenaline system either as well as, or instead of, serotonin.

Significant advantages may be claimed for some of these, but the evidence is that all antidepressants are equally effective and the decision about what drug to prescribe needs to be made on the basis of what suits the patient and their lifestyle. Antidepressants are not addictive, unlike the benzodiazepines, but withdrawal symptoms may occur if the drug is stopped suddenly.

Other drugs that may be used, especially for patients who do not respond to tricyclics, include monoamine oxidase inhibitors such as isocarboxazid (Marplan) and phenelzine (Nardil), but the older drugs in this group have potentially serious side-effects and are most often used by specialists. Lithium is used in the treatment of bipolar depression and patients require careful monitoring of blood levels.

Hypericum (St John's Wort) has been much written about in the press, is available over the counter and is very popular. It seems to have features of SSRIs and of monoamine oxidase inhibitors (MAOIs), and appears to be effective in mild to moderate depression. It is widely believed to be free of side-effects but this may not be the

Table 1. The aetiology of depression

Factor/component	Biological	Social	Psychological
Predisposing	Inheritance (especially bipolar); intrauterine damage or birth trauma; physical deprivation in childhood	Emotional deprivation in childhood; bereavement or separation; chronic problems at work; long-standing relationship difficulties; lack of other supporting relationships	Inadequate parental role models, including mental illness, alcohol/drug use; low self-esteem
Precipitating	Recent infections, for example, flu; disabling or life-threatening illness or injury	Recent loss or threat of loss; for example spouse, job or other important loss	Maladaptive responses to other factors leading to helplessness
Maintaining	Chronic pain or disability especially sensory impairment	Chronic problems relating to housing finance, work, marriage, family and friends; lack of confiding relationship; lack of information about how to deal with social problems	Low self-esteem doubts about recovery from illness; effects of long-term dependency on benefits

case. There are suggestions of food interactions similar to those experienced with the MAOIs.

Counselling is very popular and there has been an enormous growth in the number of counsellors in general practice in recent years. Until recently, there was a great deal of concern expressed about the level of training and expertise of these counsellors. The situation seems to have improved considerably, though there is still no regulatory body for the profession.

There is continuing controversy about the efficacy of counselling, which is related to the fact that it is hard to define exactly what is meant by this term. It may be the case that targeted counselling at those most likely to benefit is the best approach.

It does seem to be helpful for relationship problems, bereavement and adjustment to other major life events. Brief counselling by health visitors has been shown to improve the outcome for mothers with postnatal depression (Cox and Holden, 1994).

Cognitive therapy, also known as cognitive behavioural therapy, is said to be as effective as drugs and it may prevent relapse (Paykel and Priest, 1992). The theoretical basis of this treatment is the belief that a characteristic negative style of thinking underlies the illness, consisting of negative perceptions of self, negative interpretations of experiences and a negative view of the future. Treatment consists of helping the patient identify these automatic negative thoughts and replace them with more positive and flexible ways of thinking. Simplified techniques, which may be used in primary care settings by GPs or nurses, have been developed.

As well as encouragement to take care of their general health, many people derive a great deal of comfort from the support of fellow suffers through self-help groups.

Problem-solving help, to deal with social difficulties, may also be useful. In addition there are a number of resources available that can help patients and their families understand the illness and get the most from their treatment.

Electroconvulsive therapy is usually a treatment of last resort reserved for people who are so ill that they require hospitalisation. In a few instances it may be a treatment of choice, particularly where previous response to it has been good (Fink, 1992).

THINKING POINT

● Consider your current caseload. Do you have patients or clients who may have an unrecognised depressive illness? What might you be able to do to ensure they get help?

PART TWO

The role of the nurse

Depression is mainly an illness encountered in primary-care settings, but there may also be high rates of unrecognised depression among patients in other settings: for example, hospital wards, hospices and in residential and care homes for older people. School nurses may encounter depressed children, and occupational health nurses may meet employees with depression. People with serious, psychotic illnesses are not immune from depression, nor are people with learning disabilities.

But the key messages are that depression is a treatable condition regardless of its cause, that improved recognition and treatment of depression reduces suicide risk, and that treating depression improves quality of life for both the person involved and his or her family or carer.

GPs fail to recognise about half of those patients who present with major depression, at least at the first consultation. A further 10% will be subsequently recognised, and about half of those unrecognised will recover spontaneously. The rest are still likely to be ill and unrecognised six months later and are at risk of developing a chronic illness (Tylee, 1996). The ability of doctors to recognise depression varies widely. Though much less is known about nurses' ability to recognise the illness, some of the information from GP research could be used by nurses to improve their skills. Table 2 shows some risk factors for depression.

During the patient consultation, GPs who are good at recognising signs of depression show interest and concern, ask about home, work and family, and make use of verbal and non-verbal cues that patients give. They also have good interviewing skills, such as making more eye contact; listening without interrupting; asking open-ended questions; asking about feelings and making empathic comments (Fig 3).

Patients whose illness is recognised are more likely to be white, female, middle-aged, unemployed, bereaved or separated and to look depressed. The illness is less likely to be recognised in adolescents, young adults, older people, students, people with physical illness and people who present with physical symptoms. There may also be difficulties if patients are reluctant to consider psychological problems or if psychological cues are given late in the interview, or not at all.

Nurses should also try to develop skills for recognising signs of depression. Hook (1994) has suggested that part of the nurse's role in the consultation is to facilitate access to the doctor, perhaps as a patient's advocate. To do this effectively for the depressed patient, the nurse will need to

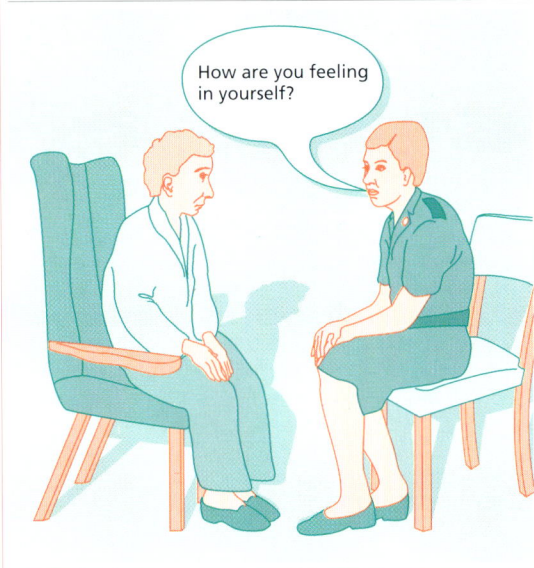

Fig 3. Open-ended questions may elicit signs of depression

> How are you feeling in yourself?

Table 2. Risk factors for depression

Bereavement
Marital or relationship problems
Family and parenting problems
Social isolation
Serious, painful, disabling or life-threatening physical illness
Sensory impairment, especially hearing or visual
Financial difficulties
Unemployment or problems at work
Housing problems
Long-term care problems
Previous history of depression

be able to outline the patient's symptoms, and to be able to help the patient understand that some of his or her unexplained symptoms might be owing to depression and that depression is a treatable illness.

SCREENING

It is possible to ask, in every patient encounter, a simple question about the way the person is feeling: 'How are you feeling in yourself?', and to follow-up any suggestion of low mood by further questions (Table 3). However, there are more formal methods of detecting mental health problems in general, and depression in particular, using screening questionnaires. Self-completion questionnaires include Hospital Anxiety and Depression Scales (HADS), validated for primary care use (Tylee, 1996); Goldberg General Health Questionnaire (GGHQ); and Edinburgh Postnatal Depression Scale (EPDS), mainly used by health visitors.

Questionnaires may be used as part of a general health assessment; for example, the Geriatric Depression Scale (GDS) has been recommended for inclusion in the over-75 health check (Katona et al, 1995). They may also be useful in audit, for example to investigate the prevalence of depression in certain groups known to be at risk. They require careful use and should be:
● Valid for the setting in which they are to be used, and appropriate for the client group
● Used only with proper explanation and patient consent
● Used in the context of a team approach with agreed interventions for people whose score indicates the presence of problems
● Used only when there is adequate back-up available for patients whose problems cannot be dealt with in the immediate setting.

Some screening tools are available through pharmaceutical company representatives or advisers. The EPDS has been published and may be copied with appropriate acknowledgements and is available in a variety of languages (Cox and Holden, 1994). Some of the most widely used scales, such as the GHQ and the HADS, are copyrighted and a fee is payable for their use.

IMPROVING TREATMENT ADHERENCE

Treatment adherence to antidepressant medication is notoriously poor. Reasons cited are poor side-effect profile and confusion in the public mind between non-addictive antidepressants and habit-forming benzodiazepines (Katona et al, 1995). These reasons tend to put the blame on the patient and ignore professional responsibility. Most authors stress the importance of a supportive atmosphere for patients. This may mean offering frequent, short appointments.

A recently published research study demonstrated that practice nurses who had received brief training were just as good as GPs at monitoring patients taking antidepressant therapy. The outcome for patients having nurse-assisted care (the intervention group) was no different from patients receiving care from their GP (the control group), though the outcome for both groups was excellent. The researchers had hoped to demonstrate that nurse-assisted care was superior to usual GP care, but the fact that control and intervention groups were in the same practices may well have meant that the GPs learnt from the nurses and improved their care too (Mann et al, 1998).

Ley has suggested that there are three main ways in which patients may be helped to get the best from their treatments (Ley 1988). These appear to go further than the methods used in the practice nurse study and, if acted on, might enhance the effects of nurse support. These are:
● Improving patient satisfaction with the consultation through listening, identifying worries and expectations
● Addressing the patient's own health beliefs
● Improving the patient's understanding and recall by avoiding jargon

- Asking for feedback
- Providing back-up written information.

PROBLEM-SOLVING AND SOCIAL SUPPORT

It is common for facilitators in primary care to encounter the attitude that says: 'First, all my patients are depressed; second, everyone around here has severe social problems; and third, I can't do anything about the problems, therefore I can't do anything about the depression.' Health professionals cannot remove all the problems experienced by their clients, but people who are severely depressed and remain untreated lack the motivation to help themselves.

There are also large numbers of patients in primary care settings whose illness does not reach the level at which drug treatment is likely to be effective but who, nevertheless, visit the doctor or nurse to ask for help. They should not be ignored. Early intervention with the most vulnerable of these people might prevent the development of a more serious, chronic illness.

Improving social support should be a common element in most interventions. Also important are enhancing problem-solving and coping skills (Murray, 1995). Professionals cannot fill the gaps for people whose social networks are poor, but they can provide information about local sources of self-help and befriending. Newton (1992) has suggested three principles to help people deal with social crises:

- Target people known to be at greatest risk. Most people will have at least one risk factor for depression but to offer support to everyone would be unmanageable and achieve little, since only those at high risk are likely to become depressed. Armstrong (1995) suggests that people with four or more risk factors might benefit from targeted help.
- Help people take control of their own lives without increasing dependency on experts. The basis of most problem-solving techniques is that people are helped to identify their problems and find solutions for themselves, with support and encouragement. Referral to helping agencies in the formal sense is not always appropriate. Empowerment means that patients are helped to make their own decisions about what is right for them, based on information that might be provided by the nurse — but the nurse does not make the decision. Moreover, the nurse continues to support the patient even though the decision may seem to the nurse to be 'wrong'.
- Make maximum use of voluntary, community and family networks and minimise use of services for people who are severely mentally ill. Experience from primary care team workshops suggests that knowledge of local sources of help and support for people in distress is generally poor. Health visitors are usually the best informed, but they are often not consulted by other members of the team. Every practice needs a working knowledge of local support agencies including advice centres, counselling organisations, self-help and support

groups and befriending agencies. A local council for voluntary service, the public library or health promotion unit may be able to supply a directory, which then needs to be kept up to date and in a place where all team members can get at it (Armstrong, 1995).

ASSESSING SUICIDE RISK

There is evidence that some suicides are preventable. Suicidal thoughts should always be taken seriously. It is a myth that people who talk about suicide do not do it, nor is it true that asking about suicide will make an attempt more likely. It is important not to dismiss all attempts at self-harm as attention-seeking. About one in 10 people who make an unsuccessful attempt will eventually succeed, many within the following year.

Most people who eventually kill themselves have some form of mental disorder, usually depression, and up to two-thirds may have seen their doctor in the previous month (Raleigh, 1996).

There are some people with depression who may be at especially high risk, including those who are socially isolated and have severe communication difficulties, in particular those who have problems sustaining interpersonal relationships.

Raised suicide rates have been noted in some ethnic minority groups, especially young Asian women and young Caribbean people, which may be indicative of widespread risk of mental disorder and self-harm (Raleigh, 1996). All patients with depression should be asked about suicidal ideas and intentions. The following questions, from the Defeat Depression Campaign *aide memoire*, may be used:

- Ideas: Do you feel that life is not worth living anymore?
- Intentions: Do you think you might act on this?
- Plans: Have you made any plans?
- Previous attempts: Have you ever tried before?

For community nurses a positive answer to any of these questions should trigger a GP referral. In particular, active plans made by someone who has survived a previous attempt should be treated very seriously and may indicate the need for urgent psychiatric referral. Assessment of suicide risk should usually only be undertaken in the context of a practice team approach, but a patient who volunteers

---

Table 3. General screening questions

How are you feeling in yourself?
Has it been interfering with your life for the past two weeks?
Have you lost interest in things?
Are you more tired than usual?
Have you lost confidence in yourself?
Do you feel guilty about things?
Do you find it difficult to concentrate?
Do you find you are not sleeping well?
Have you lost/increased your appetite/weight?
Do you feel that life is not worth living anymore?

suicidal feelings should always be referred to a doctor for further assessment. Where a doctor is not available, referral to the Samaritans, who have a national helpline, may be appropriate.

PART THREE

Professional issues

The final part of this unit on depression looks at some professional issues that may arise when general-trained nurses begin to take responsibility for caring for the whole patient, in mind as well as body.

General nurses in a variety of settings are beginning to realise that nursing education frequently fails to prepare them to help their patients and clients with mental health problems. Appropriate continuing education courses are scarce. Nurses have also complained that the courses that do exist are often irrelevant to their needs. Additionally, they report that it may be near impossible to obtain funding or to arrange release. Nurses working part-time (which is common in the community) often have to attend courses in their own time or not at all (Jenkins, 1992).

Nor is it good enough for nurses to say that mental health is solely the province of the psychiatric nurse. Psychiatric nurses are a relatively scarce resource, and are likely to be fully committed to caring for people with serious, enduring mental illness — and more than 90% of people with mental illness are treated in general practice (Jenkins, 1992). It does, however, raise the issue of working relationships between community psychiatric nurses (CPNs) and their community nurse colleagues. Nationally, there is tremendous variability in the quality of team working, both within the primary care team itself and within the nursing team.

Of crucial importance is the issue of the mental health of nurses themselves. Working with people who have mental health problems, especially asking questions about suicide, raises all kinds of spectres: of the fear of madness, which is deep rooted and from which professionals are not immune; of the stigma that still attaches to mental ill-health and which tends to isolate people with it from 'normal' society; and of episodes of mental illness or of suicide that may have arisen in the nurse's own family.

Nurses who have themselves experienced mental illness are not always treated with understanding by their professional colleagues, managers or employers. Yet it needs to be understood that the very qualities that bring a person to work in a caring profession may also make him or her vulnerable.

EDUCATION AND TRAINING

That depression can be seen as a primary care illness does not mean that GPs and community nurses have to take on a whole load of new work. The work is already there. The problem is that much depression goes unrecognised and therefore untreated. People with untreated problems are high users of practice time. At the Bath Model Practice Project, which has systematically learnt to deal more effectively with depressed and anxious people, practice staff believe that although it takes persistence in the early stages, once the recognition and treatment of these illnesses improves, life gets much better for practice staff as well as for patients.

The first national census of practice nurses estimated that about 40% were involved in the early detection of depression and anxiety (Atkin et al, 1993). In a survey covering two health districts, 89% of practice nurse respondents said they dealt with psychological problems, 87% felt inadequately trained and 91% wanted more training in mental health (Thomas and Corney, 1993). Practice nurses are in the forefront of attempts to improve this aspect of care and to influence the provision of appropriate training. Much of what follows is the result of working by and with practice nurses.

It is odd that while some GP employers appear perfectly happy for practice nurses to give neuroleptic drugs to patients with schizophrenia, they may be reluctant to concede a role for practice nurses in the management of patients with major depression. However, there is research evidence that such nurses can take on responsibility for the care and monitoring of this group of patients in cooperation with the GP (Mann et al , 1998). There is also a good deal of experience from research and development projects that shows that practice nurses, with the support

Fig 4. A three-stage approach to mental health disorders for primary care nurses

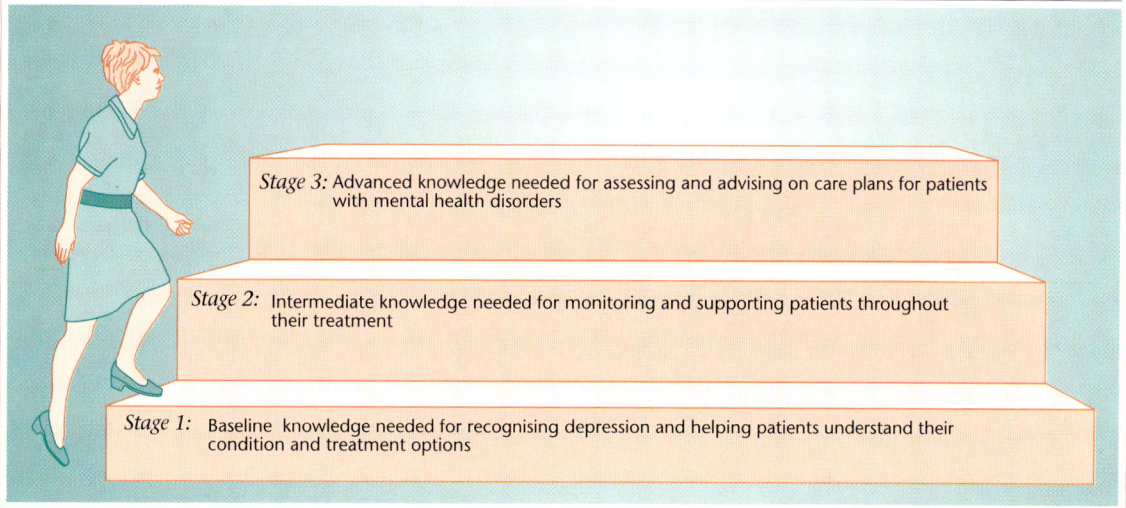

Stage 3: Advanced knowledge needed for assessing and advising on care plans for patients with mental health disorders

Stage 2: Intermediate knowledge needed for monitoring and supporting patients throughout their treatment

Stage 1: Baseline knowledge needed for recognising depression and helping patients understand their condition and treatment options

and agreement of the rest of the primary care team, can acquire the skills and knowledge to make an important contribution to the care of people with milder illnesses and psychosocial difficulties.

A focus group in London looked at the contributions nurses could make to the care of patients with common mental disorders, not just depression, given certain conditions (Armstrong, 1995). These discussions led to the development of a three-stage approach to acquiring relevant competencies.

The group felt that nurses should only take on extra responsibilities in the context of a whole team approach, and with the full agreement of colleagues. It is especially important that nurses should not routinely assess for suicide risk outside an agreed practice protocol. Nurses should not put themselves in a position where they might be left 'holding' a suicidal patient with no medical support. Access to clinical supervision (in the sense understood by counsellors) would also seem to be a prerequisite. Nurses also felt that there was a need for employers, particularly GPs, to understand nurses' professional responsibility and accountability, which means GPs responding promptly to requests for discussion about patients' care.

A THREE-STAGE FRAMEWORK (FIG 4)

In order to clarify the roles and skills of non-mental health nurses with regard to supporting people who are experiencing depression, a three-stage model can be identified with reference to the literature.

Though this framework applies to practice nurses, there is much in it which will be relevant for other general nurses. Particular groups might need to adapt it for their own needs, taking out what does not apply and adding extra things as appropriate. For example, health visitors should be familiar with the use of the Edinburgh Postnatal Depression Scale and have appropriate counselling skills. Nurses working in homes for the older people need to be aware that depression is common in such institutions. Confusion may be a symptom of depression in older people, and this needs to be distinguished from confusion caused by dementia. Depression is treatable and regimes that address boredom and isolation may be preventive. In hospital, especially in wards treating patients for life-threatening conditions such as cancer, heart disease and AIDS, awareness of the risks of depression and of the need to treat it should be high.

Stage one
This is the base line. All RGN-qualified nurses should have sufficient knowledge to be able to practise at this level. They should be able to:
● Recognises depression and refer patients appropriately
● Help patients understand their illness and the need for treatment
● Be familiar with treatment options, including medication and psychosocial interventions, and the role of the practice counsellor, if there is one
● Have a working knowledge of local advice and support agencies
● Assess suicide risk.

When making general health assessments, the nurse should be able to assess mental health, either using a screening questionnaire or by asking appropriate questions. Ideally there should be an agreed practice-wide approach to these problems. The nurse will require well-developed counselling skills and good interview technique.
Stage two
With some extra training, the nurse should be able to take on extra tasks, such as monitoring and supporting patients taking antidepressant medication, incorporating mental

health into all health promotion activities, including an assessment of risk factors for depression in all new patient health checks and other health assessments.

With practice colleagues, they can also develop a system of offering problem-solving help to high-risk, vulnerable patients and groups, build a practice library of sources of information for staff, patients and carers, including leaflets, books, audio and videotapes, and provide information and advice to patients on self-help for stress and anxiety.

Additionally, they can set up liaison with the local A&E department so that the practice is notified early whenever a patient is admitted following an episode of self-harm. This might enable the practice team to offer early support. A group of practices work with a local community mental health team to develop this kind of approach. Nurses can facilitate this sort of activity.

The extra knowledge and skills required to enable nurses to practise at this level will include:
● Knowledge of commonly used antidepressants and their side-effects (a practice prescribing policy for these drugs may be helpful)
● Risk factors for depression and suicide
● A problem-solving approach to helping people deal with social difficulties
● Stress and anxiety management techniques
● Local sources of treatment for patients with severe anxiety and phobias, for example, community psychiatric nurses and/or clinical psychologists
● Clinical audit methods for mental health.

Stage three
A nurse practising at this level would fulfil the role of mental health specialist within the team. Courses that might enable a practice nurse to practise at this level are slowly being developed but do not yet seem to be widely available. In addition to full implementation of stage two, the nurse would:
● In consultation with the GP, make full assessments of patients with depression and manage their care including follow-up of patients taking antidepressants
● Maintain records of all high-risk patients and ensure adequate support is in place
● Offer support to people wanting to withdraw from tranquilliser use
● Use cognitive interventions with depressed and anxious people
● Audit mental health care within the practice, including care of people with serious mental illness (in cooperation with key workers)
● Act as adviser to other members of the team and support nursing colleagues.

A nurse with this level of expertise might also be able to act as a mentor to nurses in other practices. He or she would need to acquire the following extra knowledge and skills:
● Clinical assessment of depression and anxiety
● Management of depression, including monitoring of antidepressant therapy
● Benzodiazepine withdrawal
● Cognitive behavioural techniques for general practice
● Working knowledge of the care programme approach (Department of Health, 1994).

TEAM WORKING

One of the clearest lessons from the above study, carried out by Mann and colleagues (1998) was that of team working . The study took place in central London from 1991 to 1994 at a time when primary care teams were poorly developed compared with other parts of the country. It was clear that the complexity of modern health care meant that in order to provide a high quality services to the public, members of the team had to recognise that no single profession had all the answers.

Community psychiatric nurses, along with other members of the community mental health team, sometimes express anxiety about general nurses taking on responsibility for mental health care, but it should be clear from this unit that the primary care of mental health is fundamentally different from the care of people with serious, enduring mental illness. Increasing the mental health skills of community nurses implies no threat to CPNs; rather, they should complement each other.

One important area where there could be cooperation between practice nurses and CPNs could be in improving physical health care for people who have a mental illness.

People with severe mental illness have higher death rates than the general population, beyond that which can be explained by higher suicide rates. They also have higher death rates from the common preventable illnesses like heart disease and cancers (Department of Health, 1994), but they are almost totally excluded from health promotion activities that are available to the general population. Engaging these people may not be easy, but it is not impossible. The greatest barrier is ignorance and stigma, as illustrated by what a receptionist said of a patient with manic depression: 'You won't get any sense out of her, she's mad.' Such attitudes should have no place in a modern health care system.

PERSONAL MENTAL HEALTH

Nurses are trained to cope. In hospital they deal not only with a rapid throughput of patients but also with the aftermath of major disasters, with highly dependant patients, and with death. In primary care there are increasing demands not only from patients, but also from administrators, often with little acknowledgement of the stress involved. Practice nurses in particular may be isolated from their peers and may have limited access to educational activities (Armstrong, 1993).

Nurses asked to identify the benefits of team work will often cite support for team members but there are dangers in believing that a well-functioning team can necessarily support all its members all the time. Teams that demand total loyalty from members may come to regard the person who seeks outside help as a traitor. Counselling services for nurses in hospital may be under-used — admitting the need for help may be interpreted as weakness by colleagues and managers, and is thought by some to lead to career 'black marks'. Against this, there is evidence that nurses with high sources of support, and satisfaction with that support, report less burnout than others, regardless of levels of stress at work (Kellet, 1991).

Accredited counsellors are required to have regular supervision which provides them with a safe environment within which difficult client problems, and their own difficulties, can be discussed with an experienced colleague. Clinical supervision for nurses is becoming more widely available and has gained acceptance within the profession. It needs to be accessible to all practitioners.

THINKING POINTS

● Do you have access to clinical or peer supervision in your area and does it meet your needs? Are there ways in which you and your colleagues could influence the way supervision is provided?
● What are the implications of the three-stage framework for your own practice? If there is no appropriate training in your area, could you and your colleagues get together to ask for it? Could your manager or practice nurse adviser help?
● What sort of contact do you have with community psychiatric nurses in your area? Is there room for improvement and could you do anything about it?

REFERENCES
Armstrong, E. (1993) Promoting mental health. In: Dines, A., Crib, A. (eds) *Health Promotion: Concepts and Practice*. Oxford: Blackwell Scientific Publications.
Armstrong, E. (1995) *Mental Heath Issues in Primary Care: A Practical Guide*. Basingstoke: Macmillan.
Armstrong, E., Tufnell, G. (1996) Childhood Depression. *Practice Nurse Journal*; 10: 243–249.
Atkin, K. et al (1993) *Nurses' Count. A National Census of Practice Nurses*. York: Social Policy Research Unit, University of York.
Cox, J., Holden, J. (1994) *Perinatal Psychiatry: Use and Misuse of the Edinburgh Postnatal Depression Scale*. London: Gaskell.
Delgado, P.L. et al (1992) *Handbook of Affective Disorders*. Edinburgh: Churchill Livingstone.
Department of Health (1994) *Health of the Nation, the Mental Illness Key Area Handbook*. London: HMSO.
Donoghue J, Tylee A. (1996) The treatment of depression: prescribing patterns of antidepressants in primary care in the UK. *British Journal of Psychiatry*; 168, 164–168.
Fink, M. (1992) Electroconvulsive therapy. In: Paykel, E.S. (ed.) *Handbook of Affective Disorders*. Edinburgh: Churchill Livingstone.
Hook, A. (1994) A framework for consultation. *Practice Nursing*; 5: 17, 37–38.
Jenkins, R. (1992) Developments in the primary care of mental illness. *International Review of Psychiatry*; 4: 237–242.
Jenkins, R. et al (1992) *The Prevention of Depression and Anxiety: The Role of the Primary Care Team*. London: HMSO, 1992.
Katona, C. et al (1995) Recognition and management of depression in late life in general practice. *Primary Care Psychiatry*; 1: 107–113.
Kellet, J. (1991) Caring about each other. *Nursing Standard*; 5: 48, 46.
Ley, P. (1988) *Communicating with Patients: Improving Communication, Satisfaction and Compliance*. London: Chapman and Hall.
Mann, A. et al (1998) An evaluation of practice nurses working with general practitioners to treat people with depression. *British Journal of General Practice*; 48. 875–879.
Meltzer, H. et al (1994) The prevalence of psychiatric disorders amongst adults aged 16–24. *Office of Population Census and Surveys: Psychiatric Morbidity in Great Britain, Bulletin No. 1*. London: OPCS.
Murray, J. (1995) *Prevention of Anxiety and Depression in Vulnerable Groups*. London: Gaskell.
Newton, J. (1992) Crisis support: utilising resources. In: Jenkins, R. et al (eds) *Prevention of Anxiety and Depression: Role of the Primary Care Team*. London: Department of Health.
Paykel, E.S., Priest, R.G. (1992) Recognition and management of depression in general practice: consensus statement. *British Medical Journal*; 305: 1198–1202.
Raleigh, V.S. (1996) Suicide patterns and trends in people of Indian subcontinent and Caribbean origin in England and Wales. *Ethnicity and Health*; 1: 1, 55–63.
Royal College of Psychiatrists (1995) *Defeat Depression Campaign: The Aspects of Depression*. London: RCP.
Thomas, R.V.R., Corney, R.H. (1993) The role of the practice nurse in mental health. *Journal of Mental Health*; 2: 65–72.
Tylee, A. (1996) The secondary prevention of depression. In: Kendrick, T. et al (eds) *The Prevention of Mental Illness in Primary Care*. Cambridge: Cambridge University Press.

Training courses

'Brief Encounters', a course for health professionals in helping patients and clients with relationship difficulties. Information from: project coordinator. One plus One, 14 Theobalds Road, London WC1N 8PF.

'The Primary Care of Mental Health — team training programme'. Information from: Ian Denson, Royal Institute of Public Health and Hygiene, 28 Portland Place, London W1N 4DE. Tel: 0171 580 2731.

Useful addresses

For information about self-help groups and other support for patients and their families, contact: Depression Alliance, PO Box 1022, London SE1 7QB.

For details of the Goldberg General Health Questionnaire and the Hospital Anxiety and Depression Scale, contact: NFER-Nelson Publishing Co. Ltd., Darville House, 2 Oxford Road East, Windsor, Berkshire.

Information about the Geriatric Depression Scale is available from Royal College of Psychiatrists, 17 Belgrave Square, London SW1X 8PG. Tel: 0171 235 2351.

Information about the Bath Model Practice Project is available from Dr George Walker, Oldfield Surgery, Upper Oldfield Park, Bath BA2 3HT.

Samaritans national helpline: 0345 909090

Depression in primary care

Assessment

When you have read the unit and completed any further reading, you can use the questions below to test your understanding of the topic. Answers can be found on the next page.

1 What proportion of people consulting their GP will have a diagnosis of major depression?

1	10%
2	90%
3	1%
4	5%

2 A client has been taking an antidepressant for the past four weeks. She is now beginning to feel better. How much longer should she continue taking the drug?

1	Four to six months
2	She can stop now
3	At least a year
4	As long as she wants

3 What is HADS?

1	A type of depression
2	A diagnostic tool
3	A screening questionnaire
4	A treatment method

4 Post-natal depression:

1	Is experienced by 10–15% of mothers
2	Is a less severe form of puerperal psychosis
3	Depends on the level of health visitor input
4	Is another name for 'baby blues'

5 Which particular 'maintaining' factor for depression puts people at serious risk?

1	Having a depressed parent
2	Virus infections
3	Low income
4	Vision and/or hearing loss

6 According to the OPCS studies, what is the most common of the neurotic disorders?

1	Sleep disorders
2	General fatigue
3	Major depression
4	Mixed anxiety and depression

7 Which of the following factors has been shown to improve doctors' recognition of depression in their patients?

1	Psychiatric training
2	Working with a counsellor
3	Making more eye contact
4	Asking more questions

8 Which of the following may explain some missed depression in patients from ethnic minorities?

1	People from ethnic minorities do not get depression
2	Most ethnic minority patients just want prescriptions
3	Cultural misunderstandings between patients and professionals
4	Ethnic minority patients can't read booklets

9 Which of the psychological treatments for depression is thought to prevent relapse?

1	Counselling
2	Gestalt therapy
3	Talking treatments
4	Cognitive therapy

10 Which of the following strategies might improve treatment adherence to antidepressants?

1	Providing back-up written information
2	Telling people they must take their drugs
3	Antidepressants don't work anyway
4	Getting relatives to check up on them

11 Which of the following conditions is most likely to run in families?

1	Major depression
2	Dysthymia
3	Bipolar depression
4	Postnatal depression

Depression in primary care

1: What proportion of people consulting their GP will have a diagnosis of major depression?
4) 5%

2: A client has been taking an antidepressant for the past four weeks. She is now beginning to feel better. How much longer should she continue taking the drug?
1) Four to six months

3: 3: What is HADS?
3) A screening questionnaire

4: Post-natal depression:
1) Is experienced by 10–15% of mothers

5: Which particular 'maintaining' factor for depression puts people at serious risk?
4) Vision and/or hearing loss

6: According to the OPCS studies, what is the most common of the neurotic disorders?
4) Mixed anxiety and depression

7: Which of the following factors has been shown to improve doctors' recognition of depression in their patients?
3) Making more eye contact

8: Which of the following may explain some missed depression in patients from ethnic minorities?
3) Cultural misunderstandings between patients and professionals

9: Which of the psychological treatments for depression is thought to prevent relapse?
4) Cognitive therapy

10: Which of the following strategies might improve treatment adherence to antidepressants?
1) Providing back-up written information

11: Which of the following conditions is most likely to run in families?
3) Bipolar depression

12: Depression is caused by:
4) A combination of biological, social and psychological factors that varies individually

13: Which of the following is a key part of offering crisis support?
1) Telling people how to solve their problems

14: What is the EPDS used for?
3) Screening for postnatal depression

ANSWERS

13 Which of the following is a key part of offering crisis support?

| 1 | Telling people how to solve their problems |
| 2 | Targeting support at the most vulnerable |

12 Depression is caused by:

1	Genetic factors
2	A traumatic event
3	Not being able to cope
4	A combination of biological, social and psychological factors that varies individually

14 What is the EPDS used for?

1	Screening for depression
2	Last resort for treatment for depression
3	Screening for postnatal depression
4	Screening for suicide risk

| 3 | Regular telephone contact |
| 4 | Referring to a counsellor |

Dementia
Knowledge for practice

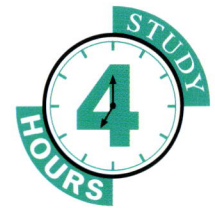

The number of people aged over 75 and the proportion they make of the total population is expected to double over the next 50 years; the number of people over 90 years is expected to increase fivefold. There are currently over 10 million older people in the UK.

It is estimated that there are 650,000 people in the UK with dementia, or 5% of people over 65. Just over half are thought to have Alzheimer's disease (Alzheimer's Disease Society, 1995a). Dementia also affects 3% of people aged 65 or under.

TYPES OF DEMENTIA

Dementia is a term that is used to describe a set of different diseases, all of which cause similar symptoms. Dementia has been defined as 'a set of symptoms where there is evidence of a decline in memory and thinking which is of a degree sufficient to impair daily living, present for six months or more' (ADS, 1995a).

Dementia causes progressive decline in a person's ability to remember, think and reason. The onset and presentation of the disease varies.

However, as it progresses, so people's ability to function and care for themselves diminishes.

Character and personality affect how people respond to changes that result from their awareness of the disease and through the organic effect on personality.

Because the progress of the disease varies from one person to another, so too does the kind of care required.

Alzheimer's disease
Alzheimer's disease is the most common form of dementia, accounting for about 50% of all cases.

It was named after Alois Alzheimer, a German neurologist who described the disease in 1906. He described the case of a 51-year old woman who had died from a mystery progressive illness. At post mortem he identified the two characteristic hallmarks of Alzheimer's disease, plaques and tangles (Fig 1 and 2).

Plaques are extra-cellular structures which consist of swollen degenerating nerve tissue. Tangles are intra-cellular structures consisting of bundles of abnormal fibres. Plaques and tangles are particularly abundant in the temporal and parietal lobes (Tobiansky, 1993). Changes also occur in the neurotransmitter system of the brain. However, research has not yet been able to identify a method to isolate this effect.

There are few known risk factors for this disease. Current research has identified that a defect on chromosome 21 may be responsible for the onset of Alzheimer's disease (Tobiansky, 1993). Aluminium levels in the blood have been linked to the development of the disease in the past. However, at present there is no conclusive evidence that

Fig 1. The brain and neuritic plaque

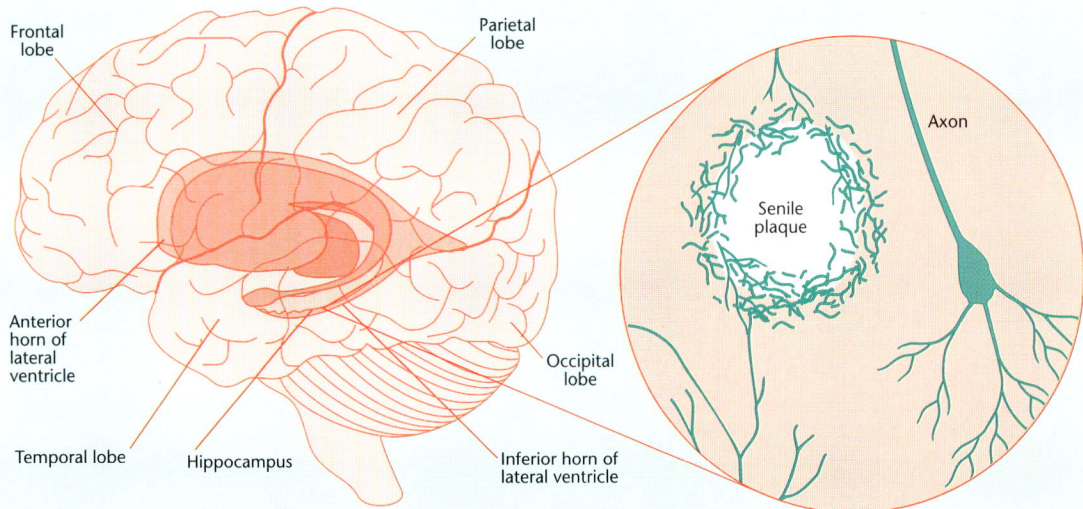

Frontal lobe
Parietal lobe
Anterior horn of lateral ventricle
Occipital lobe
Temporal lobe
Hippocampus
Inferior horn of lateral ventricle
Axon
Senile plaque

Hippocampus: One of two curved bands of a very special type of cortex, about 5cm long, on the floor of the inferior horn of the lateral ventricle on each side of the brain

DEMENTIA

Table 1. Clinical features of depression, dementia and acute confusional state			
	Dementia	*Acute confusional state*	*Depression*
Onset	Slow (months/years)	Rapid	Gradual (weeks/months)
Presentation	Alert, disoriented Poor recent memory	Fluctuating consciousness Disoriented in time, place person	Alert, worse in the mornings Oriented
Speech	Perseverative conversation	Bizarre ideas and conversation	Slow but normal content
Perception	Hallucinations in 30%, otherwise normal	Visual and auditory hallucinations	Normal, but can occasion severe depression

This chart is a guide to common presentation and should not be used exclusively for assessment and data interpretation

aluminium is a causative factor (Edwardson, 1991).

Vascular dementia

The term 'vascular dementia' has been used to describe this particular form only relatively recently. Vascular dementia used to be described as arteriosclerotic dementia. It was identified, however, that arteriosclerosis is often present in vascular dementia (Tobiansky, 1994a).

Vascular dementia is responsible for 20% of all types of dementia in Western Europe and occurs more commonly in old age. Contributing factors correspond with those risks associated with stroke and cerebrovascular disease. These include smoking, heart disease and excessive alcohol intake.

Vascular dementia is caused when small clots are carried into the cortical areas of the brain. These cause lack of oxygen to the brain and ultimate death of those particular brain cells.

The normal patterns of symptoms is that the person may present with transient ischaemic attacks, loss of eyesight, falls, confusion, dysarthria and dysphasia. Hypertension is often present (Tobiansky, 1994).

Diagnosis can sometimes be confirmed by computer tomography (CT) scan. If this type of dementia is diagnosed and the underlying cause identified it is possible to improve the person's condition through symptomatic treatment.

Lewy body dementia

This type of dementia has not been generally recognised, although it was described in 1912 by Lewy as being a result of the cortical changes observed in Parkinson's disease.

Lewy bodies are pink-staining structures found in the cytoplasm of neurones. They occur in the brain stem and cortical areas of the brain. They are present in Parkinson's disease and may be present even when dementia is not.

People with diffuse Lewy body disease or Lewy body dementia show marked impairment of parietal lobe functions: for example, they have difficulties with hand-eye coordination tasks and dyspraxia.

Dementia caused by the profusion of Lewy bodies pre-

sents in a different way to other dementias. The usual loss of memory expected in dementia is not so common. Symptoms frequently include visual or auditory hallucinations, fluctuating episodes or confusion or lucidity and unexplained falls.

Patients with Lewy body dementia often have mild forms of parkinsonism with the associated symptoms. A person with Lewy body dementia is often sensitive to psychotropic drugs which cause mild spontaneous extrapyramidal features, such as tremor in the hands. The course of the disease is variable but usually follows a pattern of deterioration interspersed with periods of stability over a period of about eight years (Livingston, 1994).

Creutzfeldt-Jakob disease (CJD)

This type of dementia has a rapid onset and prognosis is poor. It is caused by small infected proteins known as prions. In cattle similar proteins cause bovine spongiform encephalitis (BSE), but whether or not humans can contract CJD from cattle remains unclear.

The clinical feature of the illness is rapidly progressing dementia. CJD can affect anybody at any age. At present there is no treatment or cure.

Alcoholic dementia

Dementia caused through the use of alcohol, commonly known as Korsakov's syndrome, is caused by a lack of the B vitamin thiamine and presents as a reduction in memory span, confabulation (that is, patients tend to make up stories to explain things) and a reduction in awareness of time. Vitamin replacement and stopping drinking will lead to improvement. However, if alcohol has been misused for a long time, permanent brain damage can occur.

TREATABLE CAUSES OF DEMENTIA

When dealing with a person with a confusional state it is important to ensure that treatable causes do not go unidentified and untreated. The most common treatable causes of confusion are:

DEMENTIA

43

- Depression
- Acute confusional state
- Hypothyroidism
- Normal pressure hydrocephalus
- Vitamin B6 (thiamine) deficiency.

The two most common disorders to be mistaken for dementia are depression and acute confusional state. See Table 1 for clinical features of the three conditions.

Depression

When presenting as dementia, depression is sometimes called pseudodementia. Depression has an onset over weeks and characteristically there is a diurnal variation in mood, with people usually feeling more depressed in the morning. They may also experience poor concentration and agitation. Depression is common in people over 65. It can also occur in people who already have dementia (ADS, 1995a).

Acute confusional state

This usually occurs over hours or days and may be the only sign of underlying physical ill health, such as an infection. Confusion is not a diagnosis but a symptom, and with appropriate treatment of the underlying cause recovery is the most common outcome within one to four weeks.

ASSESSMENT OF A PERSON WITH DEMENTIA

A person who is admitted to any unit with symptoms that could suggest dementia should always be examined carefully to exclude other physiological reasons.

Laboratory tests should be carried out to exclude infection. The nurse should also pay careful attention to the person's dietary and fluid intake and weight to ascertain whether there are any nutritional deficiencies.

Pain can cause acute confusional problems in older people, as can the medication that may be used to alleviate it. An altered sleep pattern, with sleep deprivation, may be causing psychological and physiological changes.

Another important part of the assessment of somebody with suspected dementia is to ascertain how he or she acts when at home. A full social and functional assessment will enable the team to identify whether there are any cultural, religious, professional or social reasons for behaviour that cannot easily be understood. The pattern of a person's daily activities, along with a clear account of memory and recall, provides invaluable information to guide treatment.

Screening tests

Screening tests can be useful pointers to a diagnosis of dementia, but they cannot confirm the diagnosis. The Alzheimer's Disease Society identifies two cognitive function tests (1995):
- The abbreviated mental test score, as a rough guide to dementia, with 10 simple questions. A score of six or less suggests dementia

- The abbreviated mental state examination, a longer and more sensitive test. It has five categories and examines language, attention, recall and orientation.

It is not possible to make a firm diagnosis of dementia without a thorough multidisciplinary assessment. Moreover, it must always be acknowledged that, even if someone has already been diagnosed as having dementia, he or she may experience an exacerbation of symptoms owing to something other than deterioration caused by the dementia.

THE PROGRESS OF DEMENTIA

For some people there is little awareness of their own deterioration, while for others occasional or regular insight into the effects of the disease causes fear and uncertainty about the future.

Every person with dementia presents and progresses through the disease in a different way. This is due in part to the disease process and can be affected by other conditions. The progress of the disease can also be influenced by the style of care the person is given. Damage done by care staff to people with dementia by their attitude, actions and approach is now believed to be observable and, indeed, measurable (Kitwood, 1995).

Three stages of dementia have been identified. This approach is felt by some to be a negative form of labelling as it categorises people and the progression of their disease by the problems with which they present. However, some form of classification does help carers and relatives gauge the difficulties their relative is experiencing.

Mild dementia

Older people may show behaviour which could otherwise be attributed to old age or laziness. They may be apathetic, or unwilling to try new things, unable to adapt to change or unable to look at new, complex ideas. They may blame others when they mislay objects and become more forgetful of recent events.

Moderate dementia

Memory of the distant past is better than of recent events; patients become muddled and attempt to do things at the wrong time of day, such as going to bed at lunch-time. They may also begin to forget names and mix up family members. They may do things that appear bizarre, such as leaving the gas on, wandering at night or neglecting their personal hygiene. They may also experience visual hallucinations and other psychotic features.

Severe dementia

In the final stages of dementia people will not only experience advanced cognitive impairment, but they will be unable to use everyday objects or understand speech.

At this stage the disease will also cause physical changes, including weight loss, incontinence, bradykinesia, tremor, epileptiform seizures, rigidity, immobility and visiospatial problems.

Emotional distress

Expressions of frustration, anger, sorrow, happiness, bewilderment or aggression may all be exhibited as a result of how patients perceive themselves, the events around them and how they are treated. Supporting the emotions of somebody with dementia is made more complicated by the cognitive problems they are experiencing.

The outlook

Dementia is incurable. The average length of the disease from diagnosis is 7–10 years. It is not possible to say exactly at what stage people are in their illness, but inability to make objects has been noted to predict a rapid rate of decline (Tobiansky, 1994b).

The ultimate cause of death is often non-specific; many die of bronchopneumonia.

THINKING POINTS

● What do you know about various types of dementia, including what causes and differentiates them?
● Can you think of a scenario where a person of a different cultural background may wrongly be diagnosed as experiencing dementia?

PART TWO

The role of the nurse

Caring for somebody with dementia can be one of the most rewarding, demanding and complex types of care a nurse can give. However, the care of people with dementia requires specialist skills that may not always be available outside units dedicated to such care. This section will identify the specialist skills required to look after people with dementia, wherever they are being nursed. However, the level of expertise and degree of need will often determine the location of care.

THE NEW CULTURE OF DEMENTIA CARE

Traditionally the care of people with enduring mental health problems, including people with dementia, was derived from a centuries-old institutionalised approach that removed socially unacceptable people from society.

Since diseases causing dementia cannot be cured, it was believed that nothing could be done for patients except provide essential care such as feeding, toileting and a safe environment.

The traditional approach to dementia concentrated on people's impairments and identified their behaviour, for example, wandering and aggression, as problems that needed to be managed. The process of identifying a person's impairments and documenting the course of the disease in terms of stages of decline is a negative approach that creates an environment where nothing positive can be achieved (Kitwood, 1998).

The new culture

The new attitude and approach to the care of people with dementia centres around the person rather than the disease. People with dementia are members of the human race and have the same rights as those who care for them. The care they receive should promote and enhance their individuality and their abilities. Essential physical care is only part of what is required. Care should also reflect the individual's abilities, interests and beliefs.

The new culture of dementia care is underpinned by a positive attitude toward the person with dementia (Kitwood, 1998). If nurses see a person with dementia as somebody who is potentially aggressive, will not understand what is said, will be incontinent and will wander off, then this is reflected in the way the nurse behaves towards the individual.

Wherever nurses care for people with dementia, a central part of their practice must be to reflect on their own attitudes about the disease and try to find ways of seeing the person as someone who has special needs and not just to see the disease and the problems it causes.

The King's Fund publication *Living Well Into Old Age* (1986) provides a set of values for care professionals, which should serve as the basis for any service:
● People with dementia have the same human value as everyone else, irrespective of their degree of disability or dependence.
● People with dementia have the same varied human needs as anyone else
● People with dementia have the same rights as other citizens
● Every person with dementia is an individual
● People with dementia have the right to forms of support which do not exploit family and friends.

Nurses need to mould practice to meet the person's needs and not take the stance of thinking that the patient needs to be managed.

MANAGING THE ENVIRONMENT OF CARE

The place where we live, no matter what our age or mental stage, affects how we feel about ourselves and how we see others. The environment of an institution makes a statement about the value placed on the residents by professionals and society as a whole.

It is important the nurses are aware of the impact the environment has on the client. Establishing the practice of

Table 2. The role of the nurse in helping people with dementia

Knowledge
The disease process
The ageing process
Psychology of ageing
Interrelationship of physical and psychological functioning
Sociology of environment and relationships
Psychology of relationship formation
Drug interaction
Common physical diseases in old age
Mental Health Act 1983
NHS and Community Care Act 1990
Carers (Recognition and Services) Act 1995
Psychology of personhood and the new culture of dementia care
Sleep and the effect of disease
Knowledge of the family dynamics
Knowledge of the financial consequences on the person and their carer(s)
Group dynamics and facilitation

Skills
Assessment of physical and mental health
Counselling skills
Personal care skills
Risk assessment
Lifting and manual handling
Validation
Reality orientation
Relationship formation
General nursing skills of common diseases of old age
Managing psychiatric emergencies
Communicating skills, including understanding non-verbal communication
Providing support for carer(s)
Negotiating and collaborative working skills with other agencies
Continence assessment
Pressure risk management
Social skills
Skills in developing a positive environment
Management of sleep disturbances
The skill of empathising and being able to identify and understand the reality of the experience of dementia
Group work and facilitation

Experience
Ability to interpret the presentation of the physical and psychological presentation of the person
Understanding of the impact dementia has on the family
Ability to balance the risks and rights of the person with dementia for the benefit of the person and the community
Ability to identify precursors to distressing episodes and minimise their impact through therapeutic intervention
Ability to identify potential physical deterioration which is a result of the person's deteriorating mental health state

trying to see the situation from the patient's point of view will help in reducing the environment's negative impact on a person with dementia (Phair and Good, 1998). The environment in which care is given can be a source of stress. For someone who cannot readily understand the world around him or her new routines, new people and new language when entering hospital can cause anxiety.

For an able-bodied person the stress is unpleasant; for a person with dementia this new world, when stresses are compounded by an inability to retain new information, can result in behaviour that is viewed as confused (Stokes, 1988). For many nurses it is not possible to influence the planning or decorating of a unit in which they work. However, this does affect the atmosphere of a clinical area. Poor decoration and inadequate maintenance contribute to an air of neglect. This can lower patients' spirits and self-esteem.

Furnishings and decorations should be chosen with care. The use of plastic chairs as a precaution against incontinence, for example, is stigmatising, uncomfortable and unnecessary, given the techniques and equipment available to help people with continence problems.

Homely furniture will assist in the overall objective to create a positive environment and will help to make people more relaxed, thus reducing antisocial behaviour and the need for sedative medication (Coles, 1992).

The layout of furniture also has an impact on people and how they act. Most communication begins spontaneously, following eye contact. The most useful layout, therefore, is for chairs to be in small groups. Chairs with high wings or geriatric chairs should be avoided as they prevent eye contact (Peachment, 1997). Small tables placed in front of chairs can cause agitation and may present an accident risk if the patient does not understand why it has been placed there.

People are naturally inquisitive and this is not necessarily different for people with dementia. Wandering is a negative label, reflecting the observer's perception of the activity. The person will usually be searching for someone or something. Locked doors, therefore, cause anxiety as the person may believe that what he or she wants is behind it.

If there is no danger to the patient or others he or she should be allowed to continue exploring, being diverted or shown a route away from danger when necessary. Restraint will only cause more frustration and therefore more unhappiness and work for the staff.

THE NURSE'S ROLE IN COMMUNICATION

Communication difficulties are commonly associated with dementia and older people. Problems are usually perceived as being part of the illness. It is generally appreciated that people with dementia have difficulty understanding the world in which they live.

Failure to give people with dementia proper attention and respect contributes more to the destruction of the person than the disease itself (Kitwood, 1998). It is often the people who appear more troublesome who get the most attention, while those who are quiet are frequently ignored.

The quality of communication is often more important than the quantity. The verbal content, tone and speed of the interaction all influence the messages that are important. Nurses must be aware of their body language, as the energy and intonation of the communication will have possibly more impact on the older person than the actual words spoken.

Some key pointers to assist with communicating with people with dementia have been identified:
● Always assume that the person with dementia can understand. Never say anything within hearing distance that you do not want him or her to hear
● Use short sentences to ensure that the person does not forget the beginning of the sentence before the end is reached
● Avoid the use of jargon and the use of expressions that should not be taken literally
● If the person does not understand, be prepared to repeat the question in a different way, but try not to introduce too many new words
● When giving instructions, break down the actions into simple steps
● Ensure that the environment is conducive to imparting important information
● Maintain eye contact and give the same message with your body and face as you are giving with words
● Watch for signs of restlessness and withdraw. Do not pursue the conversation if the person is not ready
● Immediate reassurance or reward is important
● Try to state things positively rather than reinforcing the person's failure.

It should be remembered that communication involves not only how nurses communicate with patients but also how professional staff communicate with each other to ensure that information to help the patient is passed on clearly and effectively.

One of the most frustrating aspects of communication is when older people with dementia repeat the same phrase or action over and over again (a phenomenon known as perseveration). It may help to find out if they are repeating themselves because of anxiety or boredom.

Activity
Encouraging people with dementia to do things for themselves is part of the nurse's role (see Table 2). There is a real danger that people with dementia in institutional settings may experience sensory deprivation — restricted stimulation caused by limited visual stimulation, limited conversation and physical activity can all add to their problems.

Encouraging people with dementia to occupy themselves is an essential part of an individualised package of care. Up to 80% of interactions in a residential setting will be related to physical care, with most being restricted to informing or asking questions (Halberg et al, 1990).

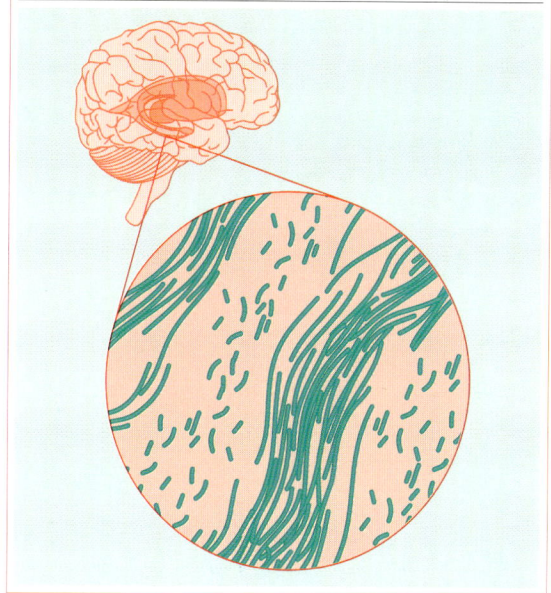
Fig 2. Neurofibrillary tangle

The caring but controlling nurse who takes a lead role in all decision-making will cause older people to do less and think less for themselves. Encouraging dependence, however well-intentioned and however unconsciously conducted, will only serve to devalue the person's self-worth and will eventually result in an increase in the care professional's workload.

Encouraging involvement in care helps the person remain physically active and prevents stiffness, muscle spasm and wasting. Activity can improve cardiac output as well as helping the person to feel valued and motivated and maintain his or her dignity.

It is important that activities have a therapeutic purpose. Stereotypical activities may include bingo, singalongs and fluffy ball-making. Other degrading scenarios include the television showing children's cartoons with the sound turned up loud or groups of old people aimlessly cutting up old Christmas cards. The nurse must discover from clients or their carers what is important to them. It may be something simple — for example, listening to The Archers on the radio or doing a jigsaw puzzle. Some people may not have any activities or hobbies that they can still manage or, indeed, they may not have had an active life in the past. None the less, carers can help identify meaningful activities for the person.

EATING WELL IN DEMENTIA

People with dementia, particularly in the latter stages, have special nutritional needs. Work has been conducted to raise awareness of staff, particularly if the person is living in residential or nursing care. Weight loss is not an inevitable consequence of dementia. The nurse should conduct appropriate assessment of the persons food intake as well as examining external factors:

- Can the person manage the utensils?
- Does any medication affect their appetite?
- Does the person have depression or constipation?
- Have they an infection?
- Are they burning up calories by moving around a lot?

Once the nurse has discovered any contributing factors they have to then identify what foods the person wants to eat and what the person recognises as enjoyable food. It is now suggested that units that do not value the social setting of eating or its impact on the whole nutritional experience may well be contributing to malnutrition or weight loss. It is now recommended that pureed foods should only be used for very specific client needs. Finger foods such as toasted tea cakes, scotch eggs or roast potatoes, can be eaten without any appearance of stigma and at the person's own pace.

If the person does need a softer diet the food can be textured, that is food that can be mashed with a fork but should not be sticky.

Making a diet interesting and enjoyable has become as aspect of care that should be offered to the highest quality and the nurse should be ensuring that catering departments in any care setting are offering what the person wants and needs (Voices, 1998).

HELPING PATIENTS EXPRESS THEIR FEELINGS

It is important to recognise the feelings of people with dementia. They retain an essential awareness, regardless of whether or not they can put it into words.

The most vital skill is to acknowledge and respond to the emotion that is being demonstrated. In order for this to be achieved, nurse and patient need to have established a relationship. Nurses must use their expertise to understand the feelings the patient is trying to express and not just rely on the words being spoken. This requires patience, understanding and professional expertise.

People with dementia sometimes become distressed by events that have happened in the past but which are very real for them now: an example might be a 90-year-old woman who is crying because her mother has just died. Try to put yourself in her position and appreciate that this pain is real for her now. The woman needs to be calmed and reassured and gently brought back to the present day. Telling her that her mother died 20 years ago and offering her a cup of tea will not alleviate her distress.

Sometimes people with dementia express their independence by refusing to do something when asked. The question should always be asked: is the request really necessary? If it is not, then patients' right to say no must be respected. If the request is necessary, rephrasing it or trying to find out why patients are reluctant to comply and dealing with the situation from their point of view is called for.

The skill of nurses is to assess, combine and use their skills, knowledge and experience in such a way that patients feel settled and content. People with dementia are often admitted into specialist units because they are presenting with aggressive, agitated behaviour, yet within a short time they have no problems. This does not happen by magic — it happens because of the skills of the nursing staff involved.

Not all nurses will have all of the skills identified. It is important that nurses recognise their own limitations and obtain assistance or seek help from a practitioner who can offer support or expert care.

THINKING POINTS

- In what ways may inappropriate care adversely affect the person with dementia?
- In what ways might the environment in which they are cared for influence the behaviour of people with dementia?
- How might you encourage a nurse who controls patients instead of helping them to act differently?
- Consider how dementia may prevent someone from giving informed consent and the implications of this for you, the nurse.

PART THREE

Professional issues

The final part of this unit on dementia considers some of the broader issues in the field. New developments in care that help people with dementia and their carers are described and the ethical implications of the disease are considered.

ETHICAL ISSUES

Nurses working with people with dementia are constantly confronted with issues that have no simple answer. People with dementia do not automatically lose their legal rights and deserve the same standards of care and degree of respect as anyone else. Patient empowerment is now commonly discussed, yet the power in making decisions depends on the patient's knowledge and ability to exercise choice (British Medical Association/RCN, 1995). Health professionals have an obligation to make every effort to provide information in an accessible manner the patient can understand.

When considering these ethical issues the philosophy for professionals should be no different from the principle that underlies all aspects of good care, that of 'do as you would be done by'.

Consent is the ability of the person to give voluntary and continuing permission of the patient based on adequate knowledge and information. As people's ability to look after themselves diminishes, it becomes difficult to avoid infringing their right to withhold consent. Promoting consent can occur in everyday situations, with decisions being made by people about what they wear and eat.

It is important to always try to obtain people's consent before doing something for them. They must, however, be able to have the capacity to understand, in simple terms, what the choice is and be able to retain the information long enough to make an effective decision. The nurse must always be aware of whether a person is able to decide to leave the building or if the decision has to be made on his or her behalf. The crucial part is that the nurse must be aware of why she undertook a particular action and what level of capacity the patient had to make the decision for himself or herself. Relatives or carers should also be involved.

Nurses must try to maintain an awareness of what level of capacity a person has to make decisions for himself or herself and try at all times to respect it. However, if treatment is necessary to safeguard life or health and wellbeing, health professionals are legally bound to give treatment without consent. If people are unable to give consent because of their continuing mental incapacity, nurses must act in their best interest.

In addition to decisions on day-to-day issues and treatment, decisions must also be made about people's financial affairs. Nurses should discuss with relatives or carers the need to take out an enduring power of attorney. This enables people with dementia to identify and name who they want to take care of their finances when they become unable to do so for themselves. If dementia has advanced to a stage where people cannot make this decision, a solicitor will have to protect their property and finances under the court of protection.

The most appropriate action for the nurse is to find out if the person has a solicitor who can deal with the problem directly. If the person does not have a legal representative the nurse should make a social work referral.

Refusing care

People have a right to refuse basic care. Nurses should try to persuade people with dementia to accept care if lack of it will lead to a deterioration of health. However, nurses must be able to justify when it is necessary to give essential personal care without consent, especially if that decision revolves around routines of the unit or personal standards rather than the patient's own wishes.

The use of restraint

The use of any form of restraint should be avoided and used only when all other forms of supporting patients have failed. Any decision to use restraint, for example, locking the unit door, putting cot sides on a bed, giving sedative drugs or putting a patient into a restraining chair, should be made only when it has been considered carefully by the multidisciplinary team and clear clinical reasons have been identified and documented.

There should be formal policies and procedures for monitoring the use of restraint. If restraint is used because of inadequate staffing, nurses have a duty to inform the relevant senior managers. Restraint is not a positive part

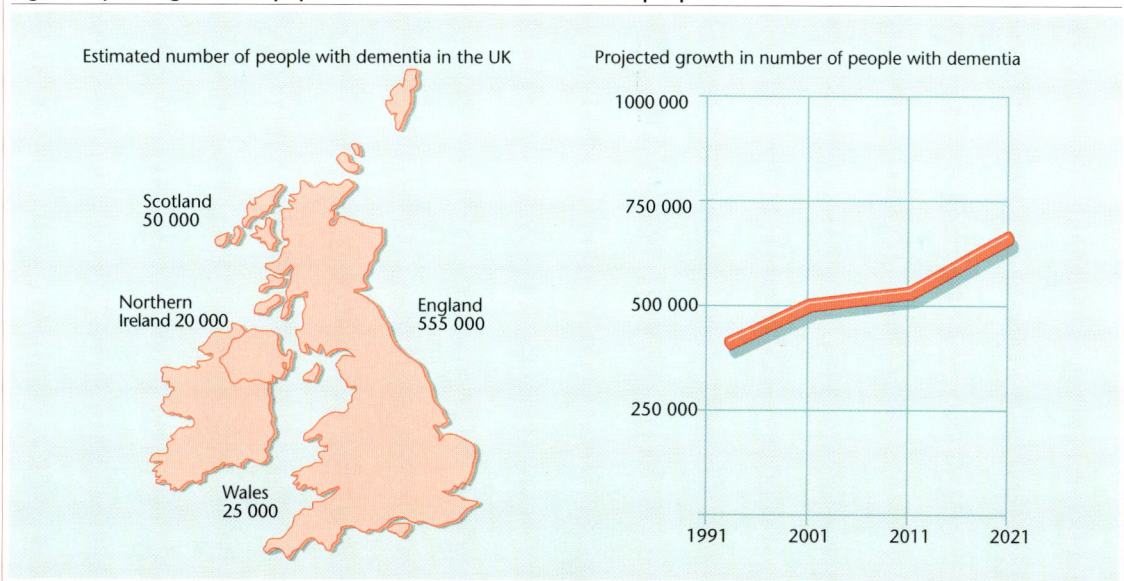

Fig 3. Projected growth in population and estimated number of people with dementia in the UK

Estimated number of people with dementia in the UK

Scotland
50 000

Northern
Ireland 20 000

England
555 000

Wales
25 000

Projected growth in number of people with dementia

1000 000

750 000

500 000

250 000

1991   2001   2011   2021

DEMENTIA

of any care package and should only ever be considered as a last resort for the shortest time possible.

SUPPORTING CARERS

It has been recognised since the Griffiths report in 1988 that those caring for people with mental health problems should receive support. This has not been forthcoming, however, across the country. The persistent failure to understand carers' needs has resulted in inappropriate, irrelevant and unavailable care.

There are four main cost areas for carers. These are financial, social, emotional and psychological, and physical costs (Scurfield, 1994). Health and social care staff have a role to play in developing methods of working to support carers and should base their work around the common areas identified by carers. These are information, skills training, emotional support and respite (Nolan and Grant, 1989).

The journey of being a carer of someone with dementia can be a lonely and tortuous one if carers and their families are not appropriately supported. The diagnosis of the disease is often uncertain and because of this carers may not be told or realise its significance immediately. For some, the diagnosis brings a slow realisation that there is something very wrong. Relatives may go to great lengths to hide the diagnosis from others because it is felt to be shameful and humiliating (Husband, 1996).

The Carer's (Recognition and Services) Act came into force in 1996. Under it each local authority is obliged to recognise and assess the needs of carers. However, access to this service varies across the UK.

Nurses should ensure that carers in their area receive the services they are entitled to and know how to gain access to an assessment. Supporting carers is an integral part of the role of the nurse in caring for people with dementia.

INNOVATION IN DEMENTIA CARE

Nurses must look at ways of supporting carers in imaginative and responsive ways in order to work towards developing a partnership with people with dementia and their families. There are a number of initiatives where nurses have worked with carers to develop ways of supporting them.

A telephone helpline service

A scheme in south-east Wales has identified the need to develop a way of supporting carers who are socially isolated (O'Donovan, 1996). The aim of the helpline is to provide carers with emotional support, information on dementia and how to gain access to specialist services, advice on welfare rights, support during a crisis and a befriending service. The scheme is coordinated by a community psychiatric nurse who takes the lead, together with a psychologist, in recruiting, training and supervising volunteers. The scheme was developed in response to a request from carers. In just two years of the scheme 1676

calls were received, thus confirming the need and indeed the value of this service.

Memory clinics

Memory clinics first appeared in the USA in the 1970s. The aim was to provide an out-patient diagnostic service and recruitment centre for people to participate in research.

The UK saw its first memory clinics in 1983 and the number has steadily grown since.

The memory clinic operates through a multidisciplinary team approach to the assessment of people who present with a memory deficit. Not only is accurate and comprehensive testing undertaken but most clinics also give advice and information to clients and their relatives, management advice and referal to Social Services if appropriate (Lindesay, 1995).

Another important aspect of their work is the ability of the clinic team to diagnose memory problems that are not due to dementia, which may have a treatable cause.

Although a diagnosis of dementia is often made when the person is referred to a psychogeriatrician for a memory problem, the emphasis of the referral may be different. Appropriate referrals to memory clinics focus on older people with a complaint of progressive memory deficit. Where there are clinics people may present earlier so the person and family can be supported by the nurse and the team from a much earlier stage in their illness.

The Admiral Nursing Service

A relatively recent development is the Admiral Nursing Service for carers of people with dementia. The aim of the service is to identify nurses who have a specific clinical role to support relatives and carers and to relieve the strain of care-giving by developing, in partnership with carers, a package of care tailored to carers' needs, which encompasses information, practical support, emotional support and skills training..

FUTURE DEVELOPMENT

The number of people with dementia is growing (Fig 3), and the role of the nurse working with these people has been highlighted as requiring complex interrelated skills, knowledge and expertise. However, the nursing role is felt by some people to be uncertain. The NHS and Community Care Act 1990 and the Department of Health eligibility criteria for NHS continuing care do not identify people with dementia as needing any significant specialist input.

In contrast to this view, the Alzheimer's Disease Society has identified that community psychiatric nurses are more useful in providing better support and information for carers than GPs (*Nursing Times*, 1995). The qualified specialist nurse does have a unique contribution to make in the care of older people. As the recognition of the potential of nursing to help people with mental health problems has grown, so care has improved, but there are still gaps in care delivery that need to be addressed. Research and education needs to be undertaken in order to develop the care of the person with dementia and the role of the nurse in that care.

There are many examples of innovative work that need to reach a wider audience. Work at the University of Wales is developing a framework to interview and work with people who have early dementia (Keady et al, 1995). The ultimate aim of the work is to establish a model of an approach to offering psychological support to the person with dementia. It is important that people in the early stages of this disease are given the opportunity to receive individualised and supportive services.

Dementia care mapping (DCM), developed by the Bradford Dementia Group, is a method of evaluating and improving the quality of care from the person's experience. It is based on detailed observation, attempting at all times to take the standpoint of the person with dementia (Kitwood and Bredin, 1994). The method bypasses many of the problems of communication by using observation as an indicator of the person's well-being or discomfort. It is founded on the philosophy already described, and this technique offers information to staff that can be used as a quality assurance tool. DCM emphasises the importance of positive personal interaction.

In busy in-patient units staff can easily become consumed with the physical care needs of patients and often ignore psychological needs. DCM helps staff identify how they are meeting the psychological needs of people with dementia.

The technique can be undertaken by anybody who has been trained in the approach. People with dementia are observed and their behaviour scored according to a validated schedule.

The scores reflect their apparent satisfaction with what is happening around them. Two mappers work together in order to validate the exercise, and information is gathered every five minutes for up to 12 hours. The data is then analysed and a care value profile, together with the patterns of care observed, form the basis for the evaluation of the care given.

DCM is not only about identifying areas of care that can be improved; it also gives staff much-needed feedback about the skills and expertise they employ regularly in their everyday practice.

In 1995 the Alzheimer's Disease Society identified the needs of younger people with Alzheimer's disease (ADS, 1995b). Seventeen thousand people below the age of 65 have the disease in the UK. The society recommends that there should be identifiable services for this client group and that the true level of need of younger people with dementia should be researched.

The last topic that should be addressed is the ability of nurses to assess and articulate their unique role in the care of this client group. Qualified and skilled nurses are needed to care for people with dementia, and the biggest challenge in the near future is to develop a clear and meaningful method to prove it.

REFERENCES

Alzheimer's Disease Society (1995a) *Dementia in the Community*. London: ADS.
Alzheimer's Disease Society (1995b) *Services for Younger People with Dementia*. London: ADS.
British Medical Association/RCN (1995) *The Older Person: Consent and Care*. London: BMA.
Coles, R. (1992) (ed) The nature of dementia with some implications for design. In: Coles R. *Signposts, Not Barriers*. Stirling: University of Stirling Dementia Services Development Centre.
Edwardson, J. (1991) Alzheimer's disease and aluminium. *Alzheimer's Review*; 1: 3, 17–22.
Halberg, I. et al (1990) A comparison between the care of vocally disruptive patients and that of other residents in psychogeriatric wards. *Journal of Advanced Nursing*; 15: 410–416.
Husband, H. (1996) Sharing the diagnosis: how do carers feel? *Journal of Dementia Care*; 14, 1, 18–20.
Keady, J. et al (1995) Listen to the voice of experience. *Journal of Dementia Care*; 12: 3, 15–17.
King's Fund Centre (1986) *Living Well Into Old Age*. London: King's Fund.
Kitwood, T. (1995) Cultures of care tradition and change. In: Kitwood, T., Benson, S. (eds) *The New Culture of Dementia Care*. London: Hawker Publications.
Kitwood, T. (1998) *Dementia Reconsidered*. Milton Keynes: Open University.
Kitwood, T., Bredin, K. (1994) Charting the course of quality care. *Journal of Dementia Care*; 4: 3, 22–23.
Lindesay, S. (1995) Memory clinics: past, present and future. *Alzheimer Review*; 5: 2.
Livingston, G. (1994) Understanding dementia: the rarer dementias. *Journal of Dementia Care*; 3: 27–29.
Nolan, M., Grant, G. (1989) Addressing the needs of informal carers: a neglected area of nursing practice. *Journal of Advanced Nursing*; 14: 930–961.
Nursing Times News (1995) CPNs better than GPs in Alzheimer care. *Nursing Times*; 91: 27, 9.
O'Donovan, S. (1995) Hold the line for carer support. *Journal of Dementia Care*; 13: 3, 20–22.
Peachment, G. (1997) You're sitting in my chair. In : Marshall, M. (ed.) *State of the Art in Dementia Care*. London: CPA.
Phair, L., Good V. (1998) *Dementia: A Positive Approach*. London: Whurr.
Scurfield, M. (1994) What do carers need? *Journal of Dementia Care*; 12: 3, 18–19.
Stokes, G. (1988) *Wandering*. Bicester: Winslow Press.
Tobiansky, R. (1993) Understanding dementia: Alzheimer's disease. *Journal of Dementia Care*; 6: 26–28.
Tobiansky, R. (1994a) Understanding dementia: vascular disease. *Journal of Dementia Care*; 1: 23–24.
Tobiansky, R. (1994b) Understanding dementia: The clinical course of dementia. *Journal of Dementia Care*; 5: 26–28.
Voices (1998) *Older People with Dementia*. Potters Bar: Voices.

FURTHER READING

British Medical Association/RCN (1995) *The Older Person: Consent and Care*. London, BMA.
Kitwood, T., Benson, S. (1995) *The New Culture of Dementia Care*. London: Hawker Publications
Phair, L., Good V. (1998) *Dementia: A Positive Approach*. London: Whurr.

Dementia

Assessment

When you have read the unit and completed any further reading, you can use the questions below to test your understanding of the topic. Answers can be found on the next page.

1 **The characteristic hallmarks of Alzheimer's disease at post mortem are:**

1	Stained structures in the cytoplasm
2	Small clots in the cortical area
3	Plaques and tangles
4	Spongy changes to the brain

2 **The most current research has identified that a cause of Alzheimer's disease may be:**

1	Linked to chromosome 21
2	Aluminium
3	Bovine spongiform encephalitis
4	Air pollution

3 **Depression that presents as dementia is sometimes called:**

1	Toxic confusional state
2	Chronic brain syndrome
3	Pseudodementia
4	Paraphrenia

4 **The patient presenting with acute confusional state may frequently be:**

1	Mentally alert
2	Drowsy in the morning but brighter in the evening
3	Unconscious
4	Showing fluctuating consciousness

5 **The use of domestic furniture in units:**

1	Helps to relax people with dementia
2	Reassures visitors of the quality of care
3	Is cost-effective
4	Can be measured positively by Dementia Care Mapping

6 **A person with dementia appears distressed and repeats a statement about her mother. Do you:**

1	Reorient her to the present
2	Divert her by offering her a cup of tea
3	Ignore her
4	Try to understand her feelings and offer support

7 **A man with dementia refuses to get undressed at bedtime. The nurse should:**

1	Inform him of his rights
2	Coerce him into getting undressed
3	Leave him be and try again later
4	Give him thioridazine to calm him down

8 **If a person is unable to give consent to care, a nurse must:**

1	Obtain permission from the next of kin
2	Act in the best interest of the patient
3	Refrain from carrying out the care
4	Ask for the patient to be detained under Section 2 of the Mental Health Act

9 **Under the Carers (Recognition and Services) Act 1995, a carer has a right to:**

1	An assessment by social services
2	Financial support
3	Respite services
4	The right to refuse care

10 **Dementia Care Mapping is a method that:**

1	Measures a person's dementia
2	Maps the care and activity of the person
3	Identifies the cost of care
4	Measures the dependency of patients

11 **If a person is unable to take care of his or her finances and has not made any arrangements, the nurse should:**

1	Ask the nearest relative
2	Ask for an assessment under the Mental Health Act
3	Ask a social worker to establish an enduring power of attorney
4	Ask a social worker to register the patient at the Court of Protection

DEMENTIA

12 An integral part of personhood is:

1	Keeping the person warm
2	Keeping the person clean and well fed
3	Engaging in positive and affirming interaction
4	Ensuring the family visit regularly

13 The NHS and Community Care Act (1990) places the responsibility of assessing the community care needs of a person with dementia with:

1	The GP
2	The community psychiatric nurse
3	Social services
4	Self-assessment by the relatives

14 Using restraint when a person is agitated:

1	Helps calm him or her down
2	May sometimes be the last resort but is not desirable
3	Is a normal part of care for people with dementia
4	Is never an option

ANSWERS

Dementia

1: The characteristic hallmarks of Alzheimer's disease at post mortem are:
3) Plaques and tangles

2: The most current research has identified that a casue of Alzheimer's may be:
1) Linked to chromosome 21

3: Depression that presents as dementia is sometimes called:
3) Pseudodementia

4: The patient presenting with acute confusional state may frequently be:
3) Unconscious

5: The use of domestic furniture in units:
3) Is cost-effective

6: A person with dementia appears distressed and repeats a statement about her mother. Do you:
4) Try to understand her feelings and offer her support

7: A man with dementia refuses to get undressed at bedtime. The nurse should:
3) Leave him be and try again later

8: If a person is unable to give consent to care, a nurse must:
1) Obtain permission from the next of kin

9: Under the Carers (Recognition and Services) Act 1995, a carer has a right to:
1) An assessment by social services

10: Dementia Care Mapping is a method that:
2) Maps the care and activity of the person

11: If a person is unable to take care of his or her finances and has not made any arrangements, the nurse should:
1) Ask the nearest relative

12: An integral part of personhood is:
3) Engaging in positive and affirming interaction

13: The NHS and Community Care Act (1990) places the responsibility of assessing the community care needs of a person with dementia with:
3) Social services

14: Using restraint when a person is agitated:
2) May sometimes be the last resort but is not desirable